Praise for The Golden Gate Diet

Finally, a voice of reason amid the cacophony of "low carb" and other fad diet "experts," advocating a scientifically sound, healthful, and practical way to lose weight. If you're ready to stop fooling yourself and start feeling better, living healthier, and looking great, take a look at the sound advice in Dr. Adam Brook's *The Golden Gate Diet*.

—*Tad Wieczorek, M.D.*
Instructor in Pathology
Harvard Medical School

Losing weight is as much a psychological challenge as it is a physical one. Adam Brook's *The Golden Gate Diet* tells you how to overcome both the physical and the psychological obstacles to losing weight. That is why *The Golden Gate Diet* works so well.

—*Jean Endicott, Ph.D.*
Professor of Clinical Psychology
Columbia University College of Physicians & Surgeons

The Golden Gate Diet is based on sound medical advice. The book is easy to read, and the diet is easy to follow. People following the Golden Gate Diet not only lose a large amount of weight, but they also reduce their risks of heart disease and stroke. This is different from low carbohydrate diets, which increase your risks of heart disease and stroke. I highly recommend the Golden Gate Diet because you will lose the weight you want to lose without risking your health.

—*Volney Sheen, M.D., Ph.D.*
Assistant Professor of Neurology
Harvard Medical School

The Golden Gate Diet tells you which foods cause cancer and which foods prevent cancer. Dr. Brook explains the medical facts clearly, in language that everyone can understand. Anyone who wants to know how to eat right should read this book.

—*James Vogel, M.D.*
Associate Clinical Professor of Medicine,
Division of Hematology and Medical Oncology
Mount Sinai School of Medicine of New York University

The Golden Gate Diet

How to Lose Weight and Maintain your Health

A Scientific Method for Weight Loss

ADAM BROOK, M.D., PH.D.

Fellow in Cardiac Surgery
Yale University School of Medicine
New Haven

Midsummer Press

Do you want to be thin and beautiful and strong?

Do you want to lose 1-2 pounds a week every week?

Do you want to cut your risk of heart disease by over 50%?

Do you want to cut your risk of cancer by 40%?

It's easy to do if you know what to eat.

This book will help you make informed decisions about how to lose weight and maintain your health. It is not a substitute for medical care by your physician. If you suspect you have a medical problem, contact your health care provider.

Design by Jennifer K. Beal

Photographs:
Page 24, aorta diseased by atherosclerosis, courtesy of T. Wieczorek, M.D., Harvard Medical School.
Page 29, bull, courtesy of C. Rahm, Natural Resources Conservation Service, United States Department of Agriculture.
Page 31, Bill Clinton, official White House Photo
Page 40, Marilyn Monroe, copyright © George Barris / MPTV.net.
Page 41, H.M. the King of Tonga, copyright © Jack Fields/CORBIS.
Page 47, Arnold Schwarzenegger, copyright © Hulton Archive/Getty images.
Page 54, apples, copyright © Jeffrey Waibel/iStockphoto.
Page 63, Inuit hunter, copyright © Staffan Widstrand/CORBIS.
Page 65, fish cartoon, copyright © The New Yorker Collection John O'Brien/cartoonbank.com. All rights reserved.
Page 68, potato cell walls, copyright © Dr. Lloyd M. Beidler/Photo Researchers, Inc.
Page 82, children with rickets, copyright © Hulton-Deutsch collection/CORBIS.

ISBN: 0-9770609-0-X

About the Author

Adam Brook graduated from Harvard College *magna cum laude* with high honors in biology. He received the M.D. degree from Harvard Medical School and the Ph.D. degree in genetics from Harvard University. He has also taught and conducted cancer research at Harvard Medical School. He trained in general surgery at Cedars-Sinai Medical Center and Mount Sinai School of Medicine-Cabrini of New York University, where he was chief surgical resident. He has been an attending general surgeon at St. Luke's Hospital in the Mission District of San Francisco. In addition to being a practicing surgeon, Dr. Brook treated patients who had difficulty losing weight or maintaining a normal weight. Dr. Brook is currently a Fellow in Cardiothoracic Surgery at the Yale University School of Medicine and the Yale-New Haven Hospital. He lectures frequently on weight loss problems.

Acknowledgments

I would like to acknowledge the following individuals for their contributions to this project.

Alise Arato, a chef with expertise in recipe development and food styling, developed the meal plans for the diet. Alise is a rising star. She has been the chef at the world-famous Aqua Day Spa. Previous clients have included Weight Watcher's®, *Wellbeing* magazine, and *Winemarket* magazine. The meals Alise developed for this book are not only so healthy, they are so good!

Ronald Goldfarb, Esq. of Goldfarb and Associates. Ron, my literary agent, has been a constant source of enthusiasm.

Jennifer Beal for a fun, hip book design. She did a beautiful job. Wendell Minor for a fascinating cover design and for his wisdom. Cheryl Waters for website design. Rachana Choubey, of Yahoo!, and Alyn Kelley, of Macromedia, for advice on technology issues. Aimée Taub, an editor at Putnam-Penguin Group, for her advice. I would also like to thank Janet Singleton, Karen Tongish, Charles Younger, Margo Silver, and Leah Zimmerman. Also, intellectual property lawyers Robert Parsons, Esq., Carol Schneider, Esq., Matthew Sant, Esq., and Roman Melnik, Esq., and entertainment lawyers Nancy Wolff, Esq., and Helene Godin, Esq.

I extend my appreciation to Andrew Muser, a talent agent at the William Morris agency.

I would like to thank my parents, Judith and David Brook, for their help and encouragement.

I would like to express my appreciation to the following physicians for their insightful comments on the diet and the manuscript:

Maurizio Daliana, M.D., Assistant Clinical Professor of Surgery, Mount Sinai School of Medicine of New York University

Jean Endicott, Ph.D., Professor of Clinical Psychology, Columbia University College of Physicians & Surgeons.

Nathan Kase, M.D., Dean Emeritus, Mount Sinai School of Medicine, formerly Chairman of Obstetrics and Gynecology, Yale University School of Medicine.

Joseph Sweeting, M.D., Professor of Clinical Medicine, Division of Digestive and Liver Disease, Columbia University College of Physicians & Surgeons.

James Vogel, M.D., Associate Clinical Professor of Medicine, Division of Hematology and Medical Oncology, Mount Sinai School of Medicine of New York University.

Badri Rengarajan, M.D., Genentech

Volney Sheen, M.D., Ph.D., Assistant Professor of Neurology, Harvard Medical School

Tad Wieczorek, M.D., Instructor in Pathology, Harvard Medical School

Warren Widmann, M.D., Associate Clinical Professor of Surgery, Columbia University College of Physicians & Surgeons.

I would also like to thank my patients for their inspiration and encouragement during all the phases of this project.

For my mother

⋆Contents⋆

Chapter 1

How to Lose Weight

and what is New about this Diet

The Golden Gate Diet is a medically sound way to lose weight. It is based
on the experiences of my patients and on the scientific literature.

I am a physician with expertise in nutrition, and my patients want to know two things
from me. First, they want to know what foods will cause them to lose weight. Second, they
want to know what foods are healthy to eat. By healthy foods, I mean foods that prevent
disease or at least do not cause disease. That is, foods that prevent heart disease and foods
that prevent cancer.

These are separate problems. Certainly many foods that will cause you to lose weight
are healthy. But there are also foods that will cause you to lose weight but will cause heart
disease. And there are even some foods—for example, nuts—that will cause you to gain
weight but are so effective at preventing heart disease that you should eat them anyway.
And, of course, there are many foods that cause you to gain weight and are very
unhealthy.

So this book answers two questions:

How do I lose weight?

What foods do I eat to stay healthy?

How do you lose weight? The key to losing weight is eating foods with a low "caloric
density."

Now this book is not hard to understand. You don't need to know any math to follow
this diet. **I have done all the math for you.**

As you will see, if you eat foods with a low caloric density, you will lose weight. If you
eat foods with a high caloric density, you will gain weight. The caloric density of any food
is a number—and that number is listed in the charts in chapter 9.

If the caloric density is less than 2, eat the food, it will help you lose weight. The lower
the number, the better.

If the caloric density is between 2 and 3, go easy.

If the caloric density is greater than 3, in general you should eat very little of that
food—it will cause you to gain weight.

You may choose to carry the chart around for the first few days. But, as you will see, it's real easy to get the hang of it. Certain groups of foods—vegetables, fruits, fish, skinless chicken, etc.—all have a low caloric density. Other groups of foods—candy, snack foods like potato chips, etc.—all have a high caloric density. My patients have had no problem in getting the hang of it quickly.

So what is caloric density?

The caloric density of a food is the number of calories in the food divided by the weight of the food.

Caloric density = calories ÷ weight

For example, chocolate pudding has a caloric density of 1.3. One half cup contains 150 calories and weighs 113 grams.

1.3 = 150 calories ÷ 113 grams

1.3 is a relatively low caloric density, so from this we know chocolate pudding is not going to ruin your diet.

In contrast, a cheese Danish has a caloric density of 3.9. One cheese Danish contains 353 calories and weighs 91 grams.

3.9 = 353 calories ÷ 91 grams

3.9 is a high caloric density, and, yes, a few cheese Danishes will ruin your diet.

Eat foods with a low caloric density, and you will lose weight.

Why does this work?

It is important to understand what makes you feel full and stop feeling hungry. While many factors go into what makes you feel full and stop feeling hungry, the most important thing is the volume of the food you are eating.

The volume of the food is the size of the food and for all practical purposes is the same as the weight of the food.* This volume of food fills up the stomach and the intestines

---

*In truth, the volume of the food is not exactly the same as the weight of the food, but it is a close enough approximation that we substitute weight for volume and get a good idea of which foods will cause you to gain weight and which foods will cause you to lose weight. In fact, for a given volume, some foods will weigh a little less than others. For example, 100 milliliters of apples weigh 64 grams. 64 grams of apples contain 38 calories, so the true caloric density of apples would be 0.4 calories per milliliter. In contrast, 100 milliliters of butter weigh 87 grams. 87 grams of butter contain 626 calories, so the true caloric density of butter would be 6.3 calories per milliliter. By these calculations butter is 16 times more fattening than apples (6.3÷0.4=16) rather than 12 times more fattening than apples, as we would have predicted from the caloric density listed in the book (7.2÷0.6=12). This is way too complicated for the purposes of this book. The caloric density as listed in this book gives you a good approximation of how fattening a food is—the higher the number, the more fattening!

and stretches the walls of the stomach and intestines.

When the walls of the stomach and intestines are stretched, the nerves in the walls of the stomach and intestines send signals to the brain—causing you to feel full and to stop feeling hungry.

For all practical purposes, two solid foods of the same volume (that is, of the same weight) will make you feel equally full and stop feeling hungry.

For example, an average-sized apple weighs 142 grams (about 5 ounces). Two and a half SNICKERS® bars also weigh 142 grams (5 ounces). Because both the apple and two and a half SNICKERS® bars weigh the same amount, whether you eat an apple or you eat two and a half SNICKERS® bars, you will basically feel equally full.

There is an important difference though!

The apple has a low caloric density. The apple has 81 calories and as we said weighs about 142 grams. The caloric density of the apple is 0.6:

$$0.6 = 81 \text{ calories} \div 142 \text{ grams}$$

The two and a half SNICKERS® bars have a high caloric density. The two and a half SNICKERS® bars have 680 calories and as we said weigh about 142 grams. The caloric density of the SNICKERS® bars is 4.8:

$$4.8 = 680 \text{ calories} \div 142 \text{ grams}$$

As we said, whether you eat an apple or you eat two and a half SNICKERS® bars, you will feel equally full, since the apple weighs as much as two and a half SNICKERS® bars. But look what's happened. If you ate the apple, you gained 81 calories. If you ate the two and a half SNICKERS® bars, you gained 680 calories!

You would have to eat about eight and a half apples to take in as many calories as there are in two and a half SNICKERS® bars.

There's no way you're eating eight and a half apples—you'll feel full long before you finish them. Believe me, it's very easy to eat two and a half SNICKERS® bars without feeling full—and two and a half SNICKERS® bars without feeling full means you just ate 680 calories without feeling full.

As you can see, if you eat apples (in reasonable quantities) you will lose weight. If you eat SNICKERS® bars you will gain weight.

That's obvious, you say. I already knew that.

While it may be obvious for apples and SNICKERS® bars, it is not always so obvious.

Cheddar cheese, which the "low carb" diets love, has a caloric density of 4.0. Don't eat it—it will cause you to gain weight.

Blueberry pie—a personal favorite of mine—has a caloric density of 2.3. Don't overdo it, but you can eat blueberry pie without ruining your diet. It is much better to eat blueberry pie than to eat chocolate cake with chocolate frosting—which has a caloric density of 3.7.

Most of my patients have lost 1-2 pounds a week on the Golden Gate Diet.

The scientific literature supports the importance of the caloric density of the food someone eats in determining their weight. A study of over 13,000 people demonstrated that the higher the caloric density of the food people ate, the heavier they were.[1]

So now that you know the principle behind losing weight, how do you eat healthily?

You will need to know some other things in addition to caloric density to eat healthily. I go over everything in detail in chapters 7 and 9. And when I say I go over everything, I mean I review everything about eating healthily. This is the latest, most up-to-date information and is based upon what I have observed from my patients as well as upon a critical review of the scientific literature.

I go over everything clearly. It won't be hard to follow. My patients have done it. You can do it.

The Golden Gate Diet will cut your risk of cancer by 40%.[2] The Golden Gate Diet will cut your risk of heart disease by over 50%.[3,4]

So even if you're not trying to lose weight, by reading this book you will learn what foods are healthy to eat. Some of it you've heard before—for example, cut down your consumption of red meat. But I think you will find some of it surprising.

This book provides you with a sample diet plan that you can use to get started. The plan lays out which foods to eat for several weeks, so that you can get an idea of how to eat right. You will be able to eat satisfying meals and have dessert too.

Did you already skip ahead to the meal plans? The meal plans were created by Alise Arato,* one of the top L.A. chefs and food stylists under 40. Alise has been the chef at the exclusive Aqua Day Spa in Santa Monica. Movie stars like Jennifer Garner go to the Aqua Day Spa to be pampered and expect to be served healthy food. Healthy cooking is what Alise is all about.

There are two meal plans: a 1200 calories a day plan for losing weight, and a 2000 calories a day plan for maintaining a low weight.

The food is so good.

Some of the foods you can have for breakfast: egg white scramble with cream cheese, cream of wheat, raspberries, blueberries, strawberries, bananas, an apricot-pineapple smoothie, oatmeal, raisin bran, Muesli cereal, French toast, waffles, pancakes (low fat of course!).

Some of the foods you can have for lunch: turkey burger, pizza with nonfat mozzarella, chicken soft tacos with low fat sour cream, tuna with mayo stuffed into tomato halves, curried chicken salad, nicoise salad with tuna and egg white, a roast beef or turkey sandwich (and I mean a proper sandwich with arugula, roasted peppers, and pesto mayo), spaghetti with chunky tomato

---

* Under my medical supervision.

sauce and cubed chicken, spinach salad with grilled shrimp and papaya, salmon salad with cucumber and herbs, turkey chili with avocado, salad with crab cake and mango salsa, Japanese soba noodle salad, a grilled Portobello sandwich with roasted peppers, baby spinach, and pesto, turkey and black bean chili, Moroccan sliced chicken breast salad with olives, figs, and orange slices, spinach salad with roasted pear and sliced grilled turkey breast, salmon burger with baby spinach, tomato, and Dijon mustard on a pita, sweet and sour chicken with vegetables.

Some of the foods you can have for dinner: braised veal chop, grilled sirloin steak with horseradish sauce, seared halibut kebabs, barbequed chicken breast (skinless of course), spaghetti with chunky tomato basil sauce, braised chicken breast, zucchini lasagna with nonfat mozzarella, pasta primavera, poached salmon with cucumber dill sauce, chicken vegetable stir fry, grilled tuna kebob with mango salsa, low fat turkey meatloaf, potato gnocchi with marinara sauce, grilled turkey breast with roasted tomato salsa, herb crusted trout with lemon, roasted chicken breast with mango salsa, grilled shrimp skewer with pineapple and bell peppers, honey orange glazed salmon, vegetable and turkey soft tacos with salsa and sour cream, grilled chicken skewers marinated in yogurt, cumin, lemon, and mint, baked red snapper with tomato, olives, and capers, baked eggplant with zucchini parmesan, linguini with white clam sauce, eye of round roast with roasted red pepper sauce.

And for dessert: a piece of blueberry, cherry, pumpkin, lemon meringue or Boston cream pie, jello, mixed berries with frozen yogurt, strawberry granita, a red wine poached pear, peach melba, grilled fruit kebab with honeyed yogurt, watermelon, fruit, apple cinnamon crumble, roasted plums, summer fruit soup, pineapple grilled with lemon and honey, citrus baked apple, chocolate, vanilla, rice, or tapioca pudding with sliced banana, angel food cake with half a sliced peach sprinkled with cinnamon, light yellow cake.

I'm getting hungry with all this writing about food and am going to go have a snack. While I'm gone, skip ahead to page 278 and look at the meals Alise has laid out. These meals are healthy! They will help you lose weight. And they taste good! Now Alise has cooked for Hollywood movie stars, but the meals she has planned are easy for you to prepare and won't take a lot of time.

I'm back. Where was I?

There are a lot of diets out there. Unfortunately they don't tell the truth. This book tells the truth and is based on scientific evidence. Because this book is based on the truth, this diet works. Most people will be able to follow this diet easily, will successfully lose weight, and will be able to keep the weight off.

The Golden Gate Diet is based on current scientific evidence using data collected using the scientific method. It was developed after a comprehensive review of the medical literature with careful review of studies of thousands of patients. It is not based on speculation or pseudoscientific mumbo jumbo as are other popular diets such as the Atkins® diet. It is based on scientific evidence and clinical experience. This diet is easy to understand and offers an approach to changing one's life.

Caloric density is the essential property that determines whether a food will help you gain or lose weight. This principle is applicable not only to this diet ("the Golden Gate Diet"), which is the ideal weight loss diet from the point of view of losing weight, but to all diets. A diet will be effective at helping you lose weight to the extent that it contains low caloric density foods. In other words, the more similar any particular diet (be it Atkins®, South Beach(tm), *etc.*) is to the Golden Gate Diet, the more effective it will be at helping you lose weight. But again, the Golden Gate Diet I have described here is the ideal diet for losing weight—it is the best possible diet for losing weight.

This diet is a healthy diet and will help you avoid heart disease and cancer—and ultimately live longer and healthier. Rather than general guidelines as to which foods help you avoid heart disease and cancer—such as are offered by the Department of Agriculture's "food pyramid"—this book tells you specifically what foods to eat to avoid heart disease and cancer.

This diet can be followed by anyone who wants to lose weight. It is not hard to do. No extreme measures are called for. You can eat satisfying, delicious foods and still stay on this diet.

You will begin this diet by eating foods with the lowest caloric density but that also taste good so that you will lose weight. You will lose 1–2 pounds a week. To lose weight faster is unhealthy. You will continue to gradually lose weight until you reach your weight goal. Then you will gradually expand what foods you eat so that you are consuming as many calories as you burn. At this point you will maintain your weight goal.

You will be encouraged to eat 3 meals a day and to eat healthy snacks 2 or 3 times a day. You will eat foods that are easy to prepare and taste good. You will not feel hungry.

You will lose weight. Yes, you will look better in a bikini. But the benefits of the diet go beyond this. You will be eating healthier. And that can help you live longer, avoid serious health problems such as heart disease, and enjoy life to its fullest. You will feel better about your body and yourself.

In addition to describing the weight loss diet, this book gives you guidelines on how to exercise—exercise is an important part of a good weight loss plan and of leading a healthy life. This book also gives you the latest information on diet drugs and weight-loss surgery. Special situations, such as smoking, diabetes, pregnancy, and overweight children are also discussed. In short, this book tells you everything you need to do to lose weight.

To summarize, this book presents you with a diet—the Golden Gate Diet—that differs from other diets:

1. The Golden Gate Diet is based on the latest medical research and on clinical evidence from actual people.
2. The Golden Gate Diet is based on the concept of Caloric Density, helping you

to limit the number of calories you eat. The Golden Gate Diet is different than the other diets that are out there. Because the Golden Gate Diet is based on the scientific principle of Caloric Density, it is easy to understand why it works. The other diets that are out there recommend you eat different foods than I recommend. For example, the Atkins® diet recommends you avoid carbohydrates, and the South Beach(tm) diet recommends you avoid foods with a high "glycemic index." In my opinion, the Atkins® and South Beach(tm) diets are not based on sound scientific principles. What matters is caloric density.

3. This diet is easy to follow and stay with. The foods I have recommended are easy to prepare and taste good. You do not have to make great sacrifices or go to extremes to stay on this diet.

This book doesn't just contain a great diet for losing weight (although it has one!) This book explains what causes someone to gain weight and what causes someone to lose weight. It also tells you which types of foods cause heart disease and cancer, and which types of foods protect against heart disease and cancer.* With this knowledge and understanding you will know how to lose weight easily and how to eat healthily.

As a scientist, physician, and surgeon I have been interested in weight problems. As a doctor I meet many people who have been trying their entire lives to lose weight. Yet there is so much confusion, misinformation, and disinformation out there about how to lose weight. With this book I clear up the confusion. I describe a diet that is easy to follow and that works. It is my deep hope that some of the people who have been trying to lose weight all their lives will read my book and achieve what they have been trying to do for so many years.

---

* I discuss which foods cause heart disease and cancer and which foods protect against heart disease and cancer in detail in chapter 7.

Chapter 2

The Weight Problem in America
and the Popular Diets that don't Work

How did I get interested in the weight problem?

The story begins in the summer after I graduated from high school. I got one of the best jobs I ever had—I worked as a timber cruiser in the Harvard forest in Petersham, Massachusetts. My friend Erik and I would hike around the woods with a compass, nail pieces of PVC pipe into the ground to mark a spot, and describe the different species of trees we saw—red maple, red oak, and the like. Petersham is a small town, so Ernie—a senior lecturer at Harvard—would drive us to the grocery in nearby Athol, and we would load up for the next two weeks.

I would head straight for the meat counter and buy 14 steaks. Every night I cooked a 16-ounce steak in a frying pan and spread butter across the top. It was the best of times.

Throughout college I didn't just eat red meat, I was a carnivore. I ate only red meat.

When I started Harvard Medical School they gave us an entrance physical where they checked some lab work. My serum cholesterol was 233. Back in those days the docs at the University Health Service didn't always measure LDL cholesterol nor were they very concerned about "modest" elevations in cholesterol—this was all just beginning. The doctor did tell me my cholesterol was at the low end of the high range and that I might think about cutting back on red meat. "You might think about getting it a little lower," he told me, "200–239 is what we call 'borderline high'."

Then, first semester of medical school, I took pathology, and they showed us a picture of an aorta—the giant artery coming out of the heart—destroyed by atherosclerotic plaque. I put two and two together and decided I had to change my ways.

I read the literature. The guidelines in force at the time called cholesterol under 200 "normal" or "desirable", with 200–239 being "borderline high" (that doesn't sound so bad, does it?). How was 200 arrived at? "Normal" cholesterol was arbitrarily defined as values below the 50th percentile on the bell-shaped curve of the general population.[5] But the literature clearly stated that the lower the cholesterol level, the lower the risk of death from coronary heart disease—even for cholesterol levels under 200! For people with "desirable" cholesterol between 182 and 202, the risk of death from coronary heart disease was found to be 29% higher than for people with a cholesterol under 182, and for people with "borderline high" cholesterol between 203 and 220, the risk of death from coronary heart disease was found to be 73% higher than for people with a cholesterol under 182.[6] To my mind, if it would be good to lower my cholesterol under 200, wouldn't it be even better if I could lower my cholesterol under 180? Why should I subject myself to a moderate risk of heart disease—assuming I could get my cholesterol down to 200—when I could have a low risk of heart disease if I got my cholesterol under 180?

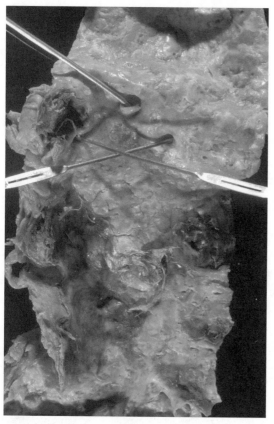

The aorta with severe atherosclerotic plaque. Courtesy of T. Wieczorek, M.D., Harvard Medical School.

I cut out red meat completely but didn't make any other changes to my diet. Maybe that would be good enough. After 6 months I had my cholesterol checked—it was down to 211. 211 was better than 233, but I wanted to see if I could get it lower.

Next I tried cutting out poultry completely. I had a notion that perhaps eating animal meats was what was causing my cholesterol to be high. Six months later I had my cholesterol checked again—still 211. They also checked my LDL cholesterol—which we now know is a better marker for heart disease risk—it was 148.

Clearly I was doing something wrong. The thing is I was eating a ton of milk products and cheese. Milk products and cheese have very high levels of saturated fat.

I started eating poultry again and eliminated all milk products and cheese, with the exception of nonfat and low fat milk products and cheese. My cholesterol plummeted to 149. My LDL cholesterol level was 94.

Of course, with the Golden Gate Diet, you'll be able to have red meat occasionally.

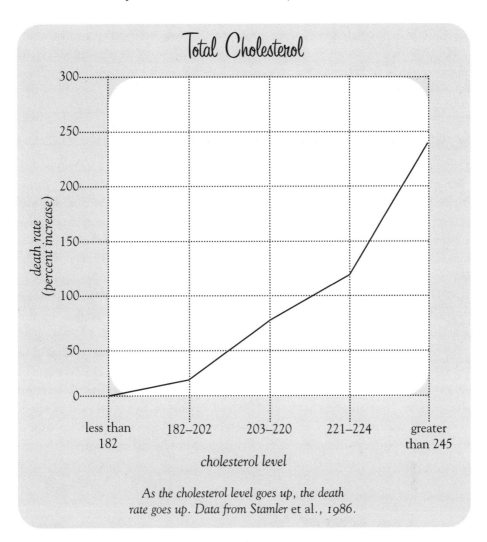

Total Cholesterol

As the cholesterol level goes up, the death rate goes up. Data from Stamler et al., 1986.

By this time I was working on my Ph.D. thesis in the Laboratory of Molecular Oncology at the Massachusetts General Hospital Cancer Center. My thesis was on molecular mechanisms of cancer, and I spent long days and nights doing molecular biology and genetics experiments in the laboratory.

During that time I did a systematic review of the literature on the causes of cancer. It turns out that the main causes of cancer in humans are not power lines, cell phones, or radio transmissions.

There are two main causes of cancer in humans—smoking and diet.

25

Specifically, a diet that is high in red meat intake leads to colon and prostate cancer.[7] Alcohol consumption causes head and neck, esophagus, liver, colon, and breast cancer.[8] And excess weight and physical inactivity also cause cancer.[9] For example, obese women have a 30% higher risk of breast cancer.[10]

So I knew about diet and heart disease, and I knew about diet and cancer.

Why would I, a surgeon, be interested in weight loss?

Surgeons think about weight all the time.

We are continually exposed to patients whose diseases ultimately are caused by their being overweight. The connection between overweight and disease requiring surgery may be direct, or the connection may be indirect. But whether direct or indirect, the connection between weight and disease is real for all the major causes of death and disability that mankind suffers: cancer, heart disease, the consequences of diabetes, and many other diseases.

In addition, certain complications of surgery, such as wound infection[11] and pulmonary embolism[12] (which is a blood clot traveling to the lungs), are far more common in overweight people than in normal weight people.

The full extent of this connection between weight and surgical disease became clear to me first when I was a surgical house officer and again when I was the chief resident.

A patient would have gangrene of the leg—which required débridement and eventually amputation. The gangrene was caused by poor circulation to the leg, which was in turn caused by atherosclerotic disease of the arteries in the leg. The atherosclerotic disease was caused by diabetes, and the diabetes was caused by being overweight.

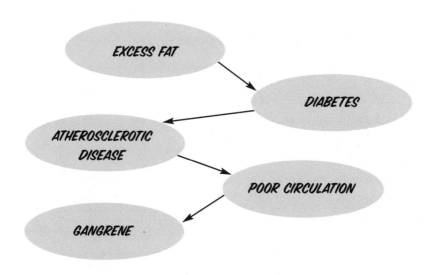

The progression could have been prevented had the patient been able to lose weight.

As an attending surgeon, I continued to find myself confronting problems of weight in my surgical patients on a daily basis. I was constantly telling my overweight patients to lose weight.

My patients would ask me how to do it. Unfortunately the diets that were out there, Atkins, Ornish, and the like, weren't working for them. Patients would lose weight, and in 6 months time they would gain all the weight back. So I developed the Golden Gate Diet.

A lot of people ask me if I have ever been very overweight and if developing the diet was some sort of personal odyssey. The truth is, I've always been thin. I am a trained scientist. Though I have never been heavy personally, I have figured out what causes people to gain weight. (You do wonder though when you hear that Dr. Atkins weighed 258 pounds.[13])

The only time I gained some weight was during residency. During the early part of residency I weighed 150 pounds. I am 5'8", so my body mass index—a measure of how heavy you are that will be discussed later—was 23—in the middle of the normal range. I went to the Elmhurst City Hospital in Queens, New York to do a trauma rotation. To my amazement, Elmhurst City Hospital—which is responsible for the health and welfare of lower-income New Yorkers—closed the hospital cafeteria and rented out the space to McDonald's®. In those days we residents slept in the hospital and put in 120 hours a week, and we had little time to eat outside of the hospital—other than going to the Mexican burrito stand down the street.

After a few months of McDonald's® and burritos my weight climbed steadily to 158 pounds. My body mass index was 24—getting towards the upper edge of normal.

Today, as an attending surgeon in California I weigh 140 pounds, and my weight is right where I want it to be. This is thanks to the Golden Gate Diet which is described in this book.

In my practice today I treat both surgical patients I operate on and non-surgical patients who come to me for help losing weight (and who don't want to become surgical patients). I have had an excellent success rate in getting patients to lose weight with the Golden Gate Diet.

The scope of the weight problem in America is vast. The National Health and Nutrition Examination Survey estimated that 64% of U.S. adults are overweight or obese.[14] In addition, 15% of children and adolescents are overweight or obese. The percentage of Americans who are very overweight has increased dramatically over the last 20 years.

The national weight problem is one of the leading public health problems in America, and many weight loss books are published every year. Many of the most popular diets do not work or are outright dangerous. A lot of people have made a lot of money feeding lies to the American public.

In particular, the Atkins® diet and other low carbohydrate diets (*e.g.* The Zone diet) are extremely popular. These diets advocate reducing carbohydrate calorie intake and support a high fat intake.[15,16] Atkins claimed for example that you gain more weight from eating 1000 calories of carbohydrates than from eating 1000 calories of fat.[17] To be blunt, this has never been proven, and what studies have been done suggest that this is not true.[18] Moreover, the Atkins® diet has never been proven to result in long-term weight loss.[19]

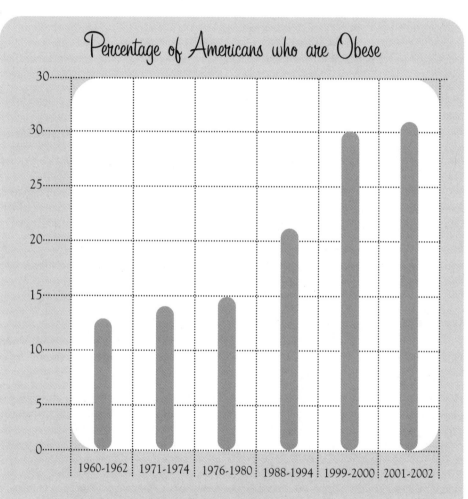

Over the last 40 years the percentage of Americans who are obese has more than doubled. Data from the National Health and Nutrition Examination Surveys 1960–1962, 1971–1974, 1976–1980, 1999–2000, and 2001–2002, which were conducted by the CDC (the Centers for Disease Control and Prevention).

What seems to be happening is that Atkins limits you to red meat, cheese, and the like. Given fewer food types to choose from, people eat less food, initially. In other words, people on Atkins initially might eat a cheeseburger without the bun rather than a cheeseburger with the bun—and a cheeseburger without the bun certainly has fewer calories than a cheeseburger with the bun, hence the initial weight loss.

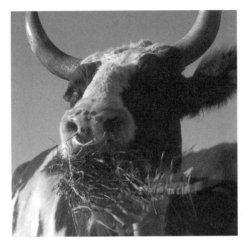

However, people like to eat different types of food—this is the way people are, and one could speculate on the reasons for this. (Of course, not all animals are like people—cattle appear to be quite content to eat grass and hay.) The vast majority of people want more variety of food choices than are available in the Atkins diet, go off the diet, and gain back all the weight they've lost.

What's worse, a high intake of animal fats has been proven to cause heart disease. This fact has been well proven in the scientific literature by multiple studies.[20,21] In fact, scientists at the Metabolic Research Group of the University of Kentucky College of Medicine and at the University of Toronto Faculty of Medicine have estimated that the Atkins® diet will increase your cholesterol on average by 51 points.[22] As we saw earlier in the chapter, an increase in your cholesterol of 51 points means an increase in your risk of heart disease of over 100%. **In my opinion, the Atkins® diet not only does not work, it can cause heart disease. Quite literally it can kill you.**

In contrast, the other extreme, the Ornish diet, preaches drastically reducing fat intake.[23] Several studies have suggested the Ornish diet may improve blood lipid profiles and help you lose weight in the short-term. It has not been proven to help you lose weight in the long-term. The major problem with the Ornish diet is that it is very difficult for patients to stick to. It is unnecessarily severe. Still, Dr. Ornish's diet is clearly in a different class than Dr. Atkins' diet: while Dr. Ornish's diet may be hard to achieve, at least it won't kill you.

Another popular diet is the South Beach(tm) diet of Dr. Arthur Agatston.[24] This diet, which is a marvel of modern marketing, advocates consumption of a diet based on low "glycemic index" foods, that is, foods that do not increase your blood sugar rapidly. In my opinion, Dr. Agatston appears to invent facts whenever it suits him. For example, in his book he states, "Numerous studies have also shown that low-glycemic foods satisfy your hunger longer and minimize your food cravings better." In fact, in 31 studies of less than 1 day, low glycemic index diets were associated with reduced hunger in 15 studies and were associated with increased hunger or no difference in hunger in 16 studies.[25] In 20 studies of less than 6 months, weight loss was seen in 4 low glycemic index diet studies and in 2 high glycemic index diet studies, and no difference between low glycemic index diets and other diets was seen in the remaining 14 studies. The average weight loss on a low glycemic index diet was about 3 pounds. There have been no good studies of the long-term effects of a low glycemic index diet. Dr. Agatston is extremely proud of his own study of 40 patients over 12 weeks. The truth is, you don't prove anything about whether a diet works long-term by looking at only 40 patients over a 12 week period.

What Atkins® and South Beach(tm) have in common is that they claim that some calories are better than other calories.

They claim that the calories from high glycemic index foods lead to weight gain but the calories from low glycemic index foods do not lead to weight gain. We have just seen that this was not found to be true in 16 of 20 studies of less than 6 months and that there are no good long-term studies. But why is this the case? The truth is that, with the exception of non-digestible fiber[26], the human body is highly efficient at absorbing almost all calories that are eaten. Perhaps this is a reflection of the many times in human history that man did not have enough food to eat[27], and so the human body became highly efficient at absorbing and incorporating all food and calories consumed. Whatever the reason, the bottom line is that once eaten, a calorie is a calorie is a calorie.

The best way to lose weight is to eat fewer calories—and the way to eat fewer calories is to eat foods that fill you up without giving you a lot of calories.

That is, the way to lose weight is to eat foods with a low caloric density.

What makes the Golden Gate Diet different from other diets is that it is based on logical scientific principles. Eating foods with low caloric density will make you feel full without taking in a lot of calories. The foods you will eat when you follow the Golden Gate Diet are different than the foods you would eat if you followed other diets. Because the Golden Gate Diet is based on scientific principles, you will lose weight, and **you will keep it off over the long run**.

Why are there so many diet books out there that not only don't work in the long run but are positively unhealthy? Why is there so much pseudo-scientific nonsense and so little truth? I am not entirely sure, but it may having something to do with the modern publishing-marketing complex. If a diet book is based on sound medical principles, it is likely to be branded as not having anything "new" and is unlikely to be published. However, if a diet book goes against sound medical principles, it can be marketed as the latest fad. This is a sad state of affairs, since people are tricked into following, for example, the Atkins diet, which is about as bad a diet as there is.

I've been told, people want to have their bacon cheeseburgers—that's why Atkins® sells so well, people want to hear that they can have their bacon cheeseburgers and still lose weight and not injure their health. If you don't care about your health, go ahead, buy Dr. Atkins' book, eat your bacon cheeseburgers. The executives at McDonald's® and Burger King® will be proud of you. But if you want to lose weight, try the Golden Gate Diet. You'll find it's not hard at all to stick to. And when you're on the beach enjoying your thin, athletic body, you'll know you've cut down your risk for heart disease and added years to your life.

President Clinton and the South Beach (tm) diet

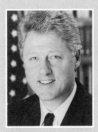

President Bill Clinton was an early advocate of the South Beach(tm) diet. He was quoted as crediting the South Beach diet for helping him lose weight.[28]

Senator Hillary Clinton worried about the diet. She told Diane Sawyer, "I didn't think it was healthy, but I know so many people who are doing that now. I'd say, 'You really think you should have a cheeseburger every day for lunch?'"

In the summer of 2004 President Clinton began developing chest pains, and he underwent quadruple coronary artery bypass surgery.

Did South Beach cause President Clinton's heart disease? The spin, if you believe the South Beach marketing machine, is that the junk food President Clinton ate before he started South Beach is what caused his heart disease. **Did the South Beach diet push him over the edge? In my opinion, it could have.**

Had President Clinton in the spring of 2003 started a low saturated fat diet like the Golden Gate Diet instead of the South Beach diet, it is unlikely he would have developed heart disease. Decreasing saturated fat intake and increasing consumption of *omega-3* fatty acids—as in the Golden Gate Diet— slows the progression of coronary artery disease and can reverse the damage that has been done to the coronary arteries.[29]

President Clinton blamed his bad diet as being the cause of his heart disease. "Since I left the White House, maybe if I had stayed on a lower fat diet. Maybe if I had ... not eaten so many hamburgers and steaks, which I love, maybe if I had, you know, had slightly less stress in my life ... maybe it would have been different."[30]

The bottom line: if you go on a "fad" low-carb diet, you are playing Russian roulette. Stay away from Atkins and South Beach. Choose a healthy diet—the Golden Gate Diet—instead.

CASE STUDY Rachel* : I lost 40 pounds in 6 months

During my first year of business school I went through a difficult break-up with my boyfriend. I relieved stress—both from the relationship and school—by eating. If I felt anxious, I would snack—potato chips, popcorn, Doritos. I am 5'4", and I got up to 170 pounds.

That winter I came down with pneumonia. I was hospitalized for 3 weeks. It was very scary—I had never been sick a day in my life before that. When you're 25 you just don't expect to get sick.

After I got out of the hospital, I decided to lead a healthier life. I was going to lose weight.

I tried the low-carb diets first. I loved the food. Who ever thought you could have steak and cheeseburgers and ice cream sundaes and still be on a diet? The problem is, I wasn't losing weight. After 2 months, I had gained 5 pounds. Plus I had been reading in the papers that low-carb diets cause heart disease. It made me nervous.

People said the low fat diets are healthy, so I tried the low fat diets. I cut out fats and basically was eating mostly vegetables. The problem is, I like food. I like to have some meat, I like to have dessert sometimes. I gave up after 2 weeks.

Then Dr. Brook recommended the Golden Gate Diet. He explained to me that the key to losing weight was eating foods that have a low caloric density.

I was surprised at how easy it is to follow. I got to eat many of the foods that I like. Chicken. Fish. Mashed potatoes! Corn. Rice. Fruit. Vegetables. Bread occasionally.

The best thing about it was I lost weight rapidly. I lost 2 pounds a week. Occasionally I would feel a little hungry, and I would have a snack. I never felt more than a little hungry.

The meals were complete and sensible. For breakfast, I could have cereal with skim milk. For lunch, a turkey sandwich and some coleslaw. For dinner, a salad, fish, spinach, corn. And I was allowed to have snacks during the day that kept me from feeling hungry.

continued..

Dr. Brook encouraged me to exercise more. I now go running 4 times a week. At first I didn't think I was going to like it, but now I like it.

It took a while, but after 6 months I had lost 40 pounds. I had reached 130 pounds.

Having reached my goal, I was able to go on what Dr. Brook calls the maintenance diet. I am now able to have very complete meals. For breakfast, sometimes I have cereal with skim milk and a banana as well or vegetarian sausages.

Sometimes pancakes. Oatmeal. Low fat waffles with syrup. An egg-white omelette with nonfat cream cheese. And sometimes I have orange juice. For lunch, I might have a turkey burger, some fruit, and nonfat pudding. Or a roast beef sandwich or pizza made with nonfat mozzarella, tomato sauce, onions, mushrooms, peppers. Who knew you could have pizza on a healthy diet! For dinner I often have chicken breast with the skin cut away or fish. Every night I have a complete meal with mashed potatoes or corn and a green vegetable. I have a glass of wine about 5 times a week. And I get to have dessert!

I understand now that caloric density is the key to weight loss. It makes sense.

I love the way my social life has improved! I am the center of attention. I have a new boyfriend, and I am much happier.

Names in case studies have been changed

Chapter 3

SOLIDS AND LIQUIDS

Are there any important exceptions to the rule that foods of equal volume make you feel equally full and stop feeling hungry? There are. A liquid food will not make you feel as full as a solid food of the same volume. This is because while solids move slowly through the stomach and intestines, liquids move rapidly through the stomach and intestines.

For a meal of a given size, liquids pass through the stomach twice as quickly as solid foods do.[31] Actually, the emptying of liquids from the stomach in comparison to solids is even faster. Liquids empty at an *exponential* rate, while solids empty at a *linear* rate. In other words, half a liquid meal might be present in the stomach after 60 minutes, but by 90 minutes none of the liquid is left in the stomach. In contrast, three-quarters of a solid meal might be present after 60 minutes, one-half of the solid meal might be present after 120 minutes, one-quarter of the solid meal might be present after 180 minutes, and not until 240 minutes would almost none of the solid meal be present in the stomach.

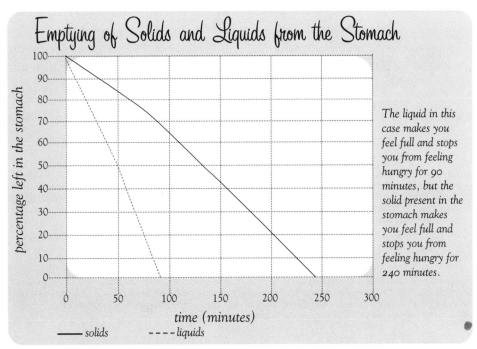

Emptying of Solids and Liquids from the Stomach

The liquid in this case makes you feel full and stops you from feeling hungry for 90 minutes, but the solid present in the stomach makes you feel full and stops you from feeling hungry for 240 minutes.

—— solids   - - - - liquids

After food leaves the stomach it enters the first part of the small intestine, which is called the duodenum. Food present in the duodenum, whether liquid or solid, also stimulates nerves traveling to the brain that give the sensation of fullness.[32] Although this has not been studied as well, it would appear that solids stimulate the duodenum to produce a feeling of fullness for a longer period of time than do liquids.*

So what is the bottom line?

Try to eat solid foods with a caloric density of 2.0 or less (the lower the caloric density, the more the food will promote weight loss).

Limit the amount of liquids that have dissolved sugars in them. In other words, avoid soda (except diet soda) and limit the amount of sweet fruit juice you drink. **In general, try to drink liquids with a caloric density of 0.4 or less. Avoid liquids with a caloric density more than 0.4.**

Foods with both a solid and a liquid component—such as most soups—are excellent for weight loss if the liquid component does not have many fats or dissolved sugars in it.† Soups (except for cream-based soups) will fill you up without giving you many calories and will help you lose weight. (But be careful if you have "sodium-sensitive" high blood pressure—many soups are high in sodium.)

When in doubt, check the tables in this book—they say clearly which foods will cause you to lose weight and which foods will cause you to gain weight.

> ### Why do some foods have a low caloric density and some foods have a high caloric density?
>
> Food is made mostly of four things: carbohydrate, protein, fat, and water. Carbohydrate and protein have about 4 calories per gram, fat has about 9 calories per gram, and water has 0 calories per gram. So foods like fruits and vegetables, which contain a large amount of water in them, have a low caloric density.

---

* It's even a little more complicated than this. Certain foods, such as bread, absorb liquid in the stomach and have a slightly greater volume in the stomach than they did before they were eaten. Other foods, for example cheese, do not absorb much liquid. So bread is slightly less fattening than its caloric density indicates, while cheese is just as fattening as its caloric density indicates. This is a minor effect, however. To be safe, to lose weight eat foods with a low caloric density and avoid foods with a high caloric density.

† And now for some bad news: ice cream and other foods that melt should be treated as a liquid. While ice cream is a solid in the freezer, as soon as it gets exposed to the 98.6 degrees body temperature in the stomach, it melts, becoming liquid. As a liquid it passes quickly out of the stomach, so it does not distend the stomach for long and does not make you feel full for long. You do burn some calories when your body heats up cold food, (such as ice cream), but this is a minor effect. If you want to lose weight, limit the amount of ice cream (and other foods that melt) that have a caloric density greater than 0.4. I'm sorry that this is not what you wanted to hear, but the truth is that if you eat a lot of ice cream, you will gain weight.

Skip ahead to chapter 9, which begins on page 94, and see what foods you can eat that will help you lose weight in a healthy way. There is a lot of variety!

Eye of round roast and braised veal cutlet, just cut the fat away. Skim milk cheeses: American, cheddar, Swiss, Muenster, cream cheese. Nonfat and 1% fat cottage cheese and yogurt, and nonfat frozen yogurt. Chicken breast and turkey white meat—cut the skin away—and egg whites and Eggbeaters. Almost every kind of fish: tuna, salmon, trout, red snapper, catfish, you name it. Every kind of shellfish: lobsters, shrimps, crabs, oysters. Every kind of fruit (except the coconut): apples, apricots, avocados, bananas, blackberries, blueberries, melons, oranges, peaches, pears, pineapple, plums, raspberries, strawberries, tangerines, watermelon. Every kind of vegetable: asparagus, broccoli, carrots, corn, onions, peppers, potatoes, squash, sweet potatoes (even candied), tomatoes. Olives and pickles. Mushrooms. Bread. Salads with low calorie dressing. Cereal: oatmeal, cream of wheat, Raisin bran. Low fat French toast, pancakes, and waffles. Pasta: macaroni, spaghetti, penne, linguini, ziti. Rice. Beans, peas, chickpeas, hummus, lentils, and tofu. Nuts and natural peanut butter. Angel food cake, light yellow cake, and Boston cream pie. All kinds of pies: apple pie, blueberry pie, cherry pie, lemon meringue pie, pumpkin pie. Puddings. Every kind of soup (except cream based soups). Ketchup, mustard, relish, and horseradish. Spices: chili powder, cinnamon, curry powder, garlic, oregano, paprika, pepper, vanilla. Light beer, white wine, and red wine.

Before you read about the Golden Gate Diet in detail, you should have a clear understanding of the reasons to lose weight. Understanding these reasons will motivate you to begin the diet and help you stick to the diet.

Chapter 4

Why Lose Weight?

Health Reasons

There are many health reasons why one should lose weight. Being overweight or obese causes or contributes to a large number of diseases, including heart disease[33,34], certain types of cancer[35], and diabetes[36]. (Body Mass Index is a way to assess whether someone is normal weight, overweight, or obese and will be discussed in the next chapter. A Body Mass Index between 19 and 24.9 is normal, and a Body Mass Index of 25 or over is overweight.)

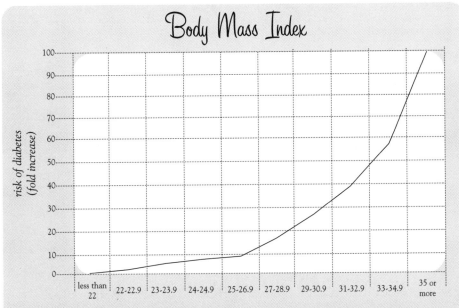

As the body mass index in women goes up, the risk of diabetes goes up.[37] A woman with a body mass index greater than 35 is 93 times more likely to have diabetes than a woman with a body mass index less than 22. Data is for non-smoking women.

Body Mass Index

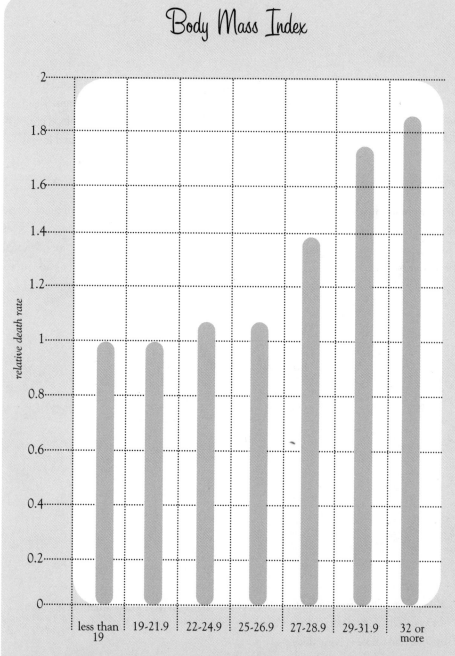

As the body mass index goes up, the death rate goes up. Data is for non-smoking women. Figure is modified from Manson *et al.*, 1995, *New England Journal of Medicine*.

In fact, it has been estimated that excess weight causes 300,000 premature deaths every year.[38] The risk of dying goes up the more overweight someone is.[39] As you can see from the chart on the opposite page, not only very overweight people have a higher death rate than people of normal weight, moderately overweight people also have a higher death rate than people of normal weight. Some of the diseases associated with being overweight are heart disease, cancer, diabetes, stroke, arthritis, breathing problems, sleep apnea, psychological disorders including depression, high blood pressure, high blood cholesterol, and gallbladder disease.[40] These diseases are associated with being sick and losing years of healthy living. They all require extensive (and expensive) medical and surgical treatments.

The life span of overweight people has been estimated to be reduced by 10%, and the life span of obese people has been estimated to be reduced by 25%.[41,42]

Overweight individuals not only live shorter lives, their lives are plagued by many illnesses. Heart disease can cause severe recurrent chest pain and debilitating shortness of breath. Diabetes can cause gangrene of the legs and kidney failure. Losing weight has been proven to lower blood pressure, lower blood glucose, and improve blood lipids.[43] These effects reduce the risk of stroke, improve diabetes, and decrease the risk of heart disease.

Overweight individuals are at higher risk for cancer of the esophagus, colon, rectum, breast, uterus, and kidney.[44]

Thus losing weight improves your health and decreases the chances of your having serious disabling diseases such as stroke, diabetes, heart disease, and cancer.

These Companies are Paying Millions to Keep you Fat

One of the strangest episodes in the American obesity epidemic is the public relations campaign being waged by America's biggest food companies to keep you fat. Under the auspices of a shadowy group called the Center for Consumer Freedom, full-page newspaper ads have appeared warning you that you are being "force-fed a steady diet of obesity myths by the 'food police,' trial lawyers, and even our own government."[45]

The Center for Consumer Freedom claims to be the champion of personal freedom. Their website states, "We believe that only you know what's best for you. When activists try to force you to live according to their vision of society, we don't take it lying down."

What the Center for Consumer Freedom wants you to believe is that it is all a myth—that there is nothing unhealthy about being overweight or obese

continued..

and that "only you know what's best for you."* You should go ahead eating French fries and hamburgers and full-fat chocolate ice cream.

Who funds the Center for Consumer Freedom? You're going to love this.

The Center for Consumer Freedom was founded in 1995 with $600,000 from Philip Morris USA Inc., the tobacco giant. Though the Center for Consumer Freedom is secretive about their funding sources, a whistleblower has revealed the names of their top contributors.* Companies such as Excel/Cargill Inc. (the leader in the beef and pork packing industry) and Wendy's each gave $200,000 to the Center for Consumer Freedom. Outback Steakhouse gave $164,000.

Who is behind the Center for Consumer Freedom?

According to the *Washington Post*, the Center for Consumer Freedom is the brainchild of Richard Berman, a Washington lobbyist and lawyer who is the center's executive director. Berman has also founded two other lobbying groups: the American Beverage Institute, which fights restrictions on alcohol use, and the Employment Policies Institute Foundation, which tries to prevent Congress from raising the minimum wage. Berman's public affairs company, Berman & Co., has received more than $7 million since 1997 from the Center for Consumer Freedom and these other groups. The Center for Consumer Freedom pretends there is a vast government conspiracy of such diverse groups as the Centers for Disease Control and Prevention, the Center for Science in the Public Interest, Mothers Against Drunk Driving, and People for the Ethical Treatment of Animals.

---

* The whistleblower told this information to the Center for Media and Democracy, a non-profit group that works to strengthen democracy by promoting media that are "of, by, and for the people."

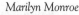

Marilyn Monroe

Social reasons

Overweight women and men are considered less attractive by many members of the opposite sex.[44,45] Obviously, a major reason why people decide to lose weight is to become more physically attractive. In our society being thin is considered the ideal. This obsession with thinness is not universal among human societies. For example, in America in the 1950s the ideal was some-

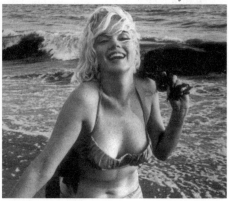

what heavier than now (witness Marilyn Monroe).

In fact, until recently a few societies considered being overweight the ideal. Up until about 20 years ago, in the island kingdom of Tonga the ideal of beauty was to be very overweight. Recently, however, the King lost weight and encouraged Tongans to become physically fit.

However, in our society being thin is considered the ideal. The purpose of this book is not to debate whether this is right or not, but to help the people who are reading this book. Because if people are thin, they can lead healthier and longer lives, can improve their self-esteem, and can improve their relationships with other people.

Overweight children are more likely to be victims of bullying than their normal weight peers.[48] This includes both "relational victimization" (withdrawing friendship or spreading rumors or lies) and "overt victimization" (name-calling, teasing, hitting, kicking, or pushing).

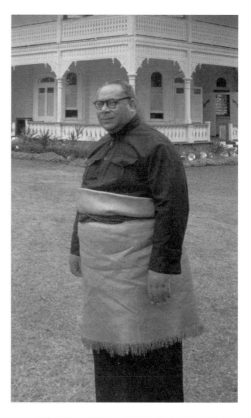

The King of Tonga H.M. Sia'osi Taufa'ahau Tupou IV

Economic Reasons

Overweight people face discrimination in the workplace. This is not limited to mean-spirited "jokes", but has been shown to have an actual dollar value associated with it. This is especially true for women, whose extra pounds translate into fewer dollars earned. A recent study demonstrated that overweight white women earned on average 5.9% less than their normal weight counterparts, and obese women earned 24.1% less than their normal weight counterparts.[49] Interestingly, only the most overweight men earned less than their normal weight counterparts.

Very overweight people are frequently denied promotions that they deserve. They are more likely to be fired and less likely to be hired because of their weight. This occurs not only in jobs where perhaps employers could make an argument that part of the job is being physically attractive (for example, fashion models), but also in jobs where one's weight should have no impact whatsoever on one's job performance!

Thus there are clear-cut dollar reasons to lose weight.

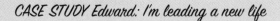

CASE STUDY Edward: I'm leading a new life

I'm a manager at a computer company in Fremont, in the Silicon Valley. My job involves setting company strategy. It's stressful, and I've put in long hours.

One day I started developing stomach pains and nausea. I've always been pretty stoic, and I thought it was heartburn. I took an antacid and decided to tough it out. But the pain didn't go away, and after four days I got a new pain that was much, much worse. It felt like being kicked in the stomach by a horse. Then I got a fever of 102 degrees and chills. I knew something was not right. I felt so sick I thought that this was it, I was done for. I went to the emergency room—that's when I met Dr. Brook.

Dr. Brook ordered a CT scan, and it turned out to be appendicitis. It was a bad case—the appendix had burst. Dr. Brook raced me to the operating room. He saved my life.

When I woke up from anesthesia I felt much better. They kept me in the hospital 5 days for intravenous antibiotics. I then went home, and after 3 weeks made a complete recovery.

Coming so close to death was a real wake-up call. I don't think it makes sense to lead the crazy, stressful life that I'd been living. I decided I wanted to work less and enjoy life more. I wanted a healthier lifestyle.

I'm a big man. I'm 6'3" tall, and at the time I weighed 250 pounds. I knew that to be healthier I needed to lose weight.

I asked Dr. Brook what to do, and he introduced me to the Golden Gate Diet.

It's a very reasonable diet. I get to eat all the healthy foods: fruit, vegetables, chicken, fish, nuts, red wine. I stay away from red meat and dairy products (unless they are nonfat). The meals are really satisfying.

continued...

I don't miss the junk food—I eat healthy snacks during the day. I do have a sirloin steak once a month as a treat. But I don't miss red meat since I can have chicken or fish instead. And I don't miss chocolate cake and cookies, since I can have other desserts—blueberry pie or angel food cake. If you're starting the diet, you need to understand that it's all about common sense—you can have a piece of blueberry pie, just don't eat the whole pie! You can have some foods that have a little higher caloric density, such as bread—just not a large amount.

I lost 30 pounds in 3 months—and I've kept the weight off.

I know 30 pounds doesn't sound like much, but boy, does it make a difference. I sleep much better at night now.

I've cut way back on the hours I put in at work. My wife and I are going to travel more this year. It's what we've always wanted to do. We just got back from a week in Paris. It was wonderful.

Chapter 5

ARE YOU OVERWEIGHT?

How do you tell if you are overweight?

You are overweight if you have a high body fat percentage. Scientists can estimate your percentage of body fat by weighing you under water (since fat is less dense than muscle and bone) or by shooting you with X-rays (since fat, muscle, and bone absorb X-rays differently).[50] These methods aren't too practical for everyday use!

The most practical good estimate of being overweight is the Body Mass Index or BMI. The actual formula for BMI is complicated! It is:

BMI=[weight (kg)]/[height(meters)]^2

Don't worry! You can figure out your BMI by using the table on the following page. Simply look for your height (in feet and inches), follow it over to your weight (in pounds), and then follow it up to the BMI scores at the top of the table on the following page.

BMI	NORMAL				OVERWEIGHT					OBESE			
	18.5	20	22	24	25	26	27	28	29	30	32	35	40
Height													
4' 10"	89	96	105	115	120	124	129	134	139	144	153	167	191
4' 11"	92	99	109	119	124	129	134	139	144	149	158	173	198
5' 0"	95	102	113	123	128	133	138	143	148	154	164	179	205
5' 1"	98	106	116	127	132	138	43	148	153	159	169	185	212
5' 2"	101	109	120	131	137	142	148	153	159	164	175	191	219
5' 3"	104	113	124	135	141	147	152	158	164	169	181	198	226
5' 4"	108	117	128	140	146	151	157	163	169	175	186	204	233
5' 5"	111	120	132	144	150	156	162	168	174	180	192	210	240
5' 6"	115	124	136	149	155	161	167	173	180	186	198	217	248
5' 7"	118	128	140	153	160	166	172	179	185	192	204	223	255
5' 8"	122	132	145	158	164	171	178	184	191	197	210	230	263
5' 9"	125	135	149	163	169	176	183	190	196	203	217	237	271
5' 10"	129	139	153	167	174	181	188	195	202	209	223	244	279
5' 11"	133	143	158	172	179	186	194	201	208	215	229	251	287
6' 0"	136	147	162	177	184	192	199	206	214	221	236	258	295
6' 1"	140	152	167	182	189	197	205	212	220	227	243	265	303
6' 2"	144	156	171	187	195	203	210	218	226	234	249	273	312
6' 3"	148	160	176	192	200	208	216	224	232	240	256	280	320
6' 4"	152	164	181	197	205	214	222	230	238	246	263	288	329
6' 5"	156	169	186	202	211	219	228	236	245	253	270	295	337
6' 6"	160	173	190	208	216	225	234	242	251	260	277	303	346

Or you can visit the Centers for Disease Control website located at
www.cdc.gov/nccdphp/dnpa/bmi/calc-bmi.htm#English

Once you've figured out what your BMI is, use the table below to determine if you are overweight and how overweight you are:

BMI

Underweight	Less than 18.5
Normal weight	18.5–24.9
Overweight	25–29.9
Obesity (class 1)	30–34.9
Obesity (class 2)	35–39.9
Extreme obesity (class 3)	40 or more

For most people the BMI is a good estimate of whether they are underweight, normal weight, overweight, or obese. Scientists have measured the percentage of body fat in different people using the X-ray technique and compared it with their BMI. This work has shown that BMI is a good but imperfect estimate of body fat.[51] Typically BMI can overestimate or underestimate the percentage of body fat by 5%.*

It is true that there are individuals who are muscular who have a high BMI. For example, when he won the Mr. Olympia contest, Arnold Schwarzenegger's height was recorded as 6' 2" tall, and his weight as 235 pounds. His BMI was 30, but he was not obese! However, this is the exceptional case. For most of us, if your BMI is high, you are probably overweight.

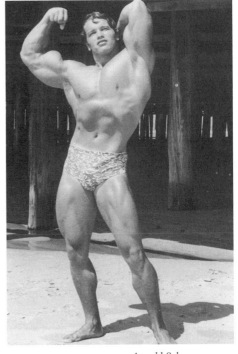

Arnold Schwarzenegger

---

* For example, people with a BMI of 20 were predicted to have a body fat percentage of 22%, but when the body fat percentages were measured more accurately using the X-ray technique, the actual body fat percentages were found to be as high as 27% or as low as 17%.

People with a BMI over 40 are candidates for weight-reduction surgery. People with diabetes or another significant weight-related illness and who have a BMI over 35 are also candidates for weight-reduction surgery.

Another measurement that should be done, in addition to BMI, is your waist circumference. Abdominal fat alone is a predictor of weight-related disease (diabetes, high blood pressure, high cholesterol, and heart disease).[52] Men with a waist circumference greater than 40 inches and women with a waist circumference greater than 35 have the same disease risk as people in the next higher BMI category who don't have a high waist circumference. For example, a woman with a BMI of 32 and a 36 inch waist has the same risk of disease as a woman with a BMI of 37 and a 33 inch waist. (And, she has a greater risk of disease than a woman with a BMI of 32 and a 33 inch waist). In other words, people with a large belly have greater health risks than people whose weight is spread throughout their bodies.*

Waist circumference should be measured not where your belt goes but at the top of the hip bones, or what doctors call the iliac crests. In other words, what doctors call "waist crcumference" is a different measurement than the measurement the salesperson in the clothing store takes when they measure your waist.

High Risk Waist Size

Women	35 inches
Men	40 inches

---

*Why does someone with a large belly have greater health risks than a person with the same BMI whose weight is spread throughout her body? Remember that BMI is just an estimate of how much fat a person has. The fat is what increases the risk of disease. For two people with the same BMI, the person with the greater waist circumference probably has more fat and less muscle and bone than the person with the smaller waist circumference. So a high waist circumference may just indicate that someone has more fat. And this idea that the fat of "apple-shaped" people is worse than the fat of "pear-shaped" people is probably just yet another fiction that has entered the popular press. In other words, for two people with the same BMI, an "apple-shaped" person probably simply has more fat and less muscle and bone than a "pear-shaped" person.

Want to gain weight? Here's how.

Crazy as it sounds, we physicians sometimes want our patients to gain weight. For example, we are operating on many patients with lung cancers, and we have much experience with patients who have had most of their stomachs removed (for example, for stomach cancer). These patients are often severely debilitated and malnourished.

How do we get our malnourished patients to gain weight? We feed them nutritional supplements, such as Ensure®, which are liquids with a high caloric density. For example, Ensure® shakes have a caloric density of 1.1, which is a high caloric density for a liquid. Because Ensure® shakes are liquid, they can pass quickly from the stomach to the intestines. In this way, they have the potential to deliver a lot of calories in patients who are unable to eat a lot of food.

What's nice about Ensure® shakes (and similar nutritional products by other companies, such as Boost®) is that they are low in saturated fat. They also provide essential vitamins and minerals, so that they can provide long-term nutrition for people needing to gain weight.

CASE STUDY Alexa: I look and feel great

I'm 25, and I work as a paralegal. Between work and my social life, I'm quite busy.

I have had to struggle to keep my weight down my whole life. I've never been very overweight. I look much better when I'm thin. The way I have dieted is by eating less. I had been down to 135 when I was seriously dieting. It just was very hard. I felt hungry all the time. After a while, I'd get busy with things, and my weight would go back up to 165.

Dr. Brook explained the Golden Gate Diet to me. It made sense. If you eat foods that will fill you up but don't have a lot of calories, you will lose weight. That's all that caloric density is about.

It was really easy to do. I didn't have to go to the grocery store and look for all kinds of crazy ingredients. I stuck to the meal plans. The meals were easy to prepare and convenient—I could have a turkey sandwich, tuna salad, or yogurt at work. I felt just a little bit hungry at times. But I lost weight fast!

I like the foods I am eating on the diet—chicken, fish, pasta, potatoes, vegetables. I feel good when I eat this food—I feel healthy. I don't miss the candy bars, the fatty cheeses, or the red meat.

Actually I lost 3 pounds a week at first. Dr. Brook says you shouldn't lose more than 2 pounds a week or you will get muscle breakdown. So I actually added other low caloric density foods to the meal plan.

That's another thing that makes sense about the diet—everyone's different. A taller person like me needs to eat more than a short person. The Golden Gate Diet says you need to individualize your diet. If you're losing weight more quickly than 2 pounds a week you should add food—low caloric density food.

When I go to the store, I read food labels. It's amazing all the bad chemicals they put in food these days. I look out for the phrase "partially hydrogenated". If it says "partially hydrogenated", it's really bad for you. It's easy to figure out the caloric density of any packaged food from the label. I try to limit the amount of food I eat that has more than 2 times as many calories as grams. At first it took a little more time to shop, but now I remember which foods have a caloric density greater than 2. It doesn't take me any more time to shop now than it did before I started the diet.

Dr. Brook says it's important to exercise. I had been embarrassed to go to the gym when I weighed 165. Not any more! I have to make a conscious effort to get to the gym since I work long hours. I try to do the Stairmaster at least half an hour a day.

I look so much better. I look much sexier!

Chapter 6

The Simple Mathematics of Calorie Reduction

What determines whether I gain weight or lose weight? The answer is simple. **If I eat more calories than I burn, I will gain weight. If I eat fewer calories than I burn, I will lose weight.**

Thus losing weight is a simple matter: **Eating fewer calories will help you lose weight. Exercising more will help you lose weight.**

Remember, if you exercise more but also eat more, you might not lose weight! I will talk about exercise more in a later chapter.

How do I eat fewer calories?

A little math here: the number of calories you eat is equal to the weight of food that you eat multiplied by the caloric density of the food.

(Calories) = (weight of food) x (caloric density)

What is "caloric density"? "Caloric density" is the number of calories in a food divided by the weight of the food. A small amount of food with high caloric density will have the same number of calories as a large amount of food with low caloric density.

How the body tells when we are full is fairly complicated. However, one key component of fullness is the amount of food we eat.

Thus, the way to eat fewer calories is:

#1 To eat foods with low caloric density. Eating a reasonable amount of foods with low caloric density is part of a healthy diet.
#2 To reduce the size of the portions of food you eat.

This is the crucial part of this diet, so I will repeat it again: **the way to eat fewer calories is:**

#1 To eat foods with low caloric density. Eating a reasonable amount of foods with low caloric density is part of a healthy diet.
#2 To reduce the size of the portions of food you eat.

Of course, one can become obese by eating a huge amount of food of low caloric density. One of my surgical colleagues told me about a patient of his who got to 450 pounds by sitting next to a bucket of apples all day long and continually eating the apples.

How do you tell which foods have low caloric density? Don't panic! Included in this book are tables listing which foods have low caloric density—and which foods to eat and which foods not to eat.

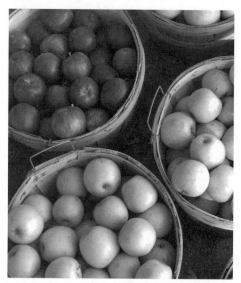

Does this mean you can only eat a few types of food? No! Be sure to check the tables for the details, but here are some of the foods you can have: Cereals. Pancakes. Egg whites prepared the way you like them. Fruit. Low fat yogurt. Salads. Soups. Bread in moderation. Nonfat cheese. Fish. Chicken and turkey, just cut the fat away. Even certain cuts of red meat such as eye of round roast and braised veal occasionally. Pasta. Rice. Corn. Potatoes. Beans. Peas. Vegetables. Nuts and natural peanut butter once you're on the maintenance phase of the diet. Puddings. Pies. Certain types of cakes. Skim milk. Juices in moderation. Diet soda. Coffee. Tea. Even a glass of wine or light beer once a day once you're on the maintenance stage of the diet. Again, it's good to check the tables, since you can't have every type of cereal, you can't have every type of cake, *etc.*

In fact, the fact that you can have many different types of food is critical. For any diet to work in the long run, you must be able to eat many different types of enjoyable food. Otherwise you won't stick to the diet. Humans crave variety in food. It's in our nature.

In addition to eating the right foods, it is important to change how you eat. Eat only during meal times. Eat 3 meals a day: breakfast, lunch, and dinner. Eat 2 or 3 snacks a day so that you will not be hungry between meals: one snack between breakfast and lunch, one snack between lunch and dinner, and (if desired) one late snack. Do not keep food nearby at other times. *Do not keep high-calorie snack foods (potato chips, pretzels, popcorn) around during work or while you are watching television.* Your snacks should be healthy foods such as a piece of fruit (an apple, a banana, or some berries), a yogurt, a low fat pudding, or a vegetable (carrots, tomatoes, green peppers).

If you are not hungry, don't eat. Don't feel obliged to finish everything on your plate. It is better to waste food than to ruin your health.

In a similar vein, parents should not force their children to eat when their children are not hungry or to clean their plates. It is better to waste food than to compromise your child's health.

CASE STUDY Nicole: As I got older I put on weight

When I was young, I was thin. As the years passed, I gained a few pounds each year. Suddenly, when I was 50 years old, I looked in the mirror and saw that I had become overweight.

I felt self-conscious about how I looked.

Then my doctor told me that I had to have surgery and that it was important for me to lose weight.

I had never been on a diet before, and the thought of it did not please me.

I decided to go on the Golden Gate Diet because it seemed the most sensible diet around.

To my surprise, the Golden Gate Diet was easy to follow. I was particularly happy that I never felt hungry on it.

I would make egg white omelettes for breakfast. I would put different vegetables in the omelette every day so it would stay interesting. Sometimes I would put in onions, sometimes mushrooms, sometimes peppers, sometimes tomatoes. I always put in a small amount of low fat cheese.

For lunch, I would have a large salad with low-calorie salad dressing. I would have it with tuna fish. Or I would have nonfat cheese on pita with tomatoes. For dessert at lunch I would have jello.

For dinner, I would have salad, eye of round roast or sirloin steak or skinless chicken, baked potatoes with low fat sour cream, and vegetables. For dessert I would have plums.

Within a short period of time I lost the weight that the doctor felt was appropriate. My surgery took place without complications.

I enjoyed the diet so much that after the surgery I decided to stay on it and move to the maintenance stage. In the maintenance stage, which I follow to this day, I have a lot more food. I always have a complete meal with salad, meat, chicken, or fish, potatoes or corn, green vegetables, and pudding or pie for dessert. I have a glass of red wine almost every day.

I am delighted with the way I look. I've had to buy new clothes, but that's been fun too. I seem to be getting more praise at work. My children are very proud of me and never fail to compliment me on how well I've done.

Chapter 7

It is Important not only to Lose Weight, but to Eat Healthy Foods as Well

Losing weight is important, but it is not the only thing! To my mind, it makes no sense to follow a diet in which you lose weight but sacrifice your long-term health. And of course, you have to be able to enjoy what you are eating!

Eating any food with a low caloric density will cause you to lose weight. But there are some foods that have a relatively low caloric density that are very unhealthy. Consider for example the egg, which the low-carb folks love. Eggs have a caloric density of 1.5, so eating eggs will not cause you to gain weight. However, 2 eggs weigh only 100 grams but contain 3.2 grams of saturated fat. They won't fill you up but will give you a large amount of saturated fat, and eating saturated fat leads to heart disease. So eggs are not a recommended food in the Golden Gate Diet, which includes only foods that both will cause you to lose weight and are healthy. (Egg whites are great though: they have a caloric density of 0.5 and contain no saturated fat.)

Saturated Fat and Cholesterol

You should limit your intake of saturated fats and cholesterol. Instead, eat unsaturated fats.

A diet low in saturated fat and cholesterol reduces the risk of heart disease and stroke. This has been well proven by many studies conducted by many different doctors.[53] Heart disease is the number one killer in the United States, and you can reduce the likelihood of heart disease and extend your lifespan by eating less saturated fat. By avoiding saturated fats you will also decrease the number of calories you are eating, since fat has 9 calories per gram.

Saturated fats cause heart disease. Monounsaturated and polyunsaturated fats protect against heart disease.[54] *Omega*-**3 fatty acids are especially effective in protecting against heart disease.[55, 56]**

Red meat is high in saturated fats. This includes beef (*i.e.* steak, hamburger, *etc.*) and pork.

What are saturated fats? Fats are made of carbon atoms in a chain. Attached to the carbon atoms are hydrogen atoms. The number of hydrogen atoms attached to the carbon atoms is different in different fats. The term "saturated" refers to the fact that carbon atoms in saturated fats have many hydrogen atoms attached to them.

What are unsaturated fats? Unsaturated fats are fats for which the carbon chains have fewer hydrogen atoms attached to them than the saturated fats do. Instead, these fats have "double bonds" between at least two of their carbon atoms.

There are two types of unsaturated fats—monounsaturated fats and polyunsaturated fats.

Monounsaturated fats are unsaturated fats with carbon chains that contain a single double bond.

Polyunsaturated fats are unsaturated fats with carbon chains that contain more than one double bond.

An important type of polyunsaturated fat is called *omega*-3 fatty acid. "Omega", the last letter in the Greek alphabet, is how chemists name the last carbon in the carbon backbone of fatty acids. "*Omega*-3" means that these fatty acids have their last double bond between the 3rd and 4th carbons from the end of the fatty acid backbone.

Poultry has a fair amount of saturated fats, although less than beef. Much of the saturated fats in poultry can be removed by cutting the skin off.

Fish have a small amount of saturated fats and a large amount of unsaturated fats. Fish is a particularly good source of *omega*-3 fatty acids. A number of excellent large studies have shown that people who eat fish on a regular basis have a lower risk of dying of heart disease.[57] My advice: **eat fish *at least* once a week.** Eating fish more than once a week is probably even better. (But read the section on mercury! A few fish are not healthy to eat. This book will tell you which fish to eat.)

Eggs are high in cholesterol and saturated fats. They are in many, many foods. Egg whites and egg substitutes (for example, Eggbeaters), however, are not high in cholesterol and saturated fats and can be used instead.

Milk (except for skim milk) is high in saturated fats. Even so-called reduced-fat milk is high in saturated fats. Most milk products are very high in saturated fats. This includes cheese, butter, and yogurt. Even reduced-fat cheese has a fair amount of saturated fats. Only nonfat cheese and nonfat yogurt have no saturated fats.

Nuts contain large amounts of monounsaturated fats and polyunsaturated fats. Nuts are a good vegetarian source of *omega-3* fatty acids. Nuts do have a high caloric density, so they are probably not the best food to eat when you are losing weight. However, once you have lost the weight you want to lose and are maintaining a stable weight, you should have 5–10 ounces of nuts a week—this will lower your risk of heart disease about 30–45%.[58]

Vegetables such as corn and vegetable oils contain large amounts of polyunsaturated fats. Olives and avocados contain monounsaturated fats. Feel free to eat corn, vegetable oils, olives, and avocados—they are all healthy foods. Soy and its products, such as tofu, are good vegetarian sources of *omega*-3 fatty acids.[59] Other vegetarian sources of *omega*-3 fatty acids include canola oil and flaxseed.[60, 61]

As it turns out, cholesterol is transported in the blood in several different types of particles. One of these particles is called low density lipoprotein (LDL), and cholesterol within the LDL particle is called LDL cholesterol.

The cholesterol in LDL particles traveling through the bloodstream can react with oxygen, a process called oxidation.[62] Oxidized cholesterol is toxic and causes inflammation. This inflammation causes LDL particles to be taken up by the walls of arteries. Once in the walls of arteries, the inflamed LDL particles and toxic oxidized cholesterol cause damage to the arterial wall—this is the process of atherosclerosis. The uptake of LDL particles into the arterial wall pushes the arterial wall into the passageway for blood, narrowing the passageway, thereby decreasing the flow of blood in the passageway.

Blood clots form on the surfaces of damaged, inflamed arteries, causing blockages.

Blocked arteries in the heart cannot supply oxygen and nutrients to the heart muscle, which then dies, causing a heart attack. Blocked arteries leading to the brain cannot supply oxygen and nutrients to brain tissue, which then dies, causing a stroke.

The way to reduce your risk of heart disease is to lower your LDL cholesterol. Lowering your LDL cholesterol will also reduce your risk of stroke.

You can lower your LDL cholesterol level by avoiding foods that are high in saturated fats and by eating foods that are high in unsaturated fats.[63] Why saturated fats increase your LDL cholesterol level and unsaturated fats lower your LDL cholesterol is not understood.

All adults aged 20 years or older should have their doctor measure a fasting lipoprotein panel every 5 years.[64] The fasting lipoprotein panel, a blood test, measures your total cholesterol, LDL cholesterol, HDL cholesterol, and triglyceride levels.

What is the ideal LDL cholesterol level? An LDL cholesterol level less than 100. If your LDL cholesterol is less than 100, you have the lowest risk of heart disease. The chart below lists different LDL cholesterol levels.[65]

LDL Cholesterol

Less than 100	optimal
100-129	above optimal/ near optimal
130-159	borderline high
160-189	high
More than 190	very high

What is the take-home message? **If your LDL cholesterol level is 130 or higher, decrease the amount of red meat and fat-containing milk products you eat.** This will lower your risk of heart disease. You should also have a discussion with your doctor if your LDL cholesterol is over 130.

In order to have the lowest risk of heart disease, decrease the amount of red meat and fat-containing milk products you eat so that your LDL cholesterol level drops below 100. This may be difficult for some people to do, and getting your LDL cholesterol level in the 100–129 range is certainly an improvement over having an LDL cholesterol over 160.

If your LDL cholesterol is high, and you are unable to lower it by diet, you may need to take cholesterol-lowering medication. Discuss this with your doctor. And if you have a history of heart disease, talk with your doctor.

A word of caution. As doctors have found that dropping the LDL cholesterol below 100 reduces the risk of heart disease, some doctors are asking if an even lower LDL cholesterol level, below 70, would be even better, especially for patients with heart disease.[66] Clearly an LDL cholesterol of 100 is better than 130, but is an LDL cholesterol of 70 better than 100? We don't know yet. Clinical trials studying this question are in progress.

While the LDL particle can cause heart disease, interestingly, a different particle, the high density lipoprotein (HDL) particle, is protective against heart disease.[67] The cholesterol in HDL particles is called HDL cholesterol. HDL cholesterol particles can remove cholesterol from artery walls[68]—cholesterol that was deposited by inflamed, oxidized LDL cholesterol particles. By removing cholesterol from artery walls, HDL stops the atherosclerotic process. HDL may also have anti-inflammatory and anti-oxidant properties.[69, 70] The higher your level of HDL cholesterol, the more effectively cholesterol is removed from your artery walls, and the lower your risk of heart disease.

People with HDL cholesterol levels below 40 are at higher risk for heart disease.[71] People with HDL cholesterol levels above 60 are at lower risk for heart disease.

The two most important factors in causing a low HDL cholesterol level are your genetic make-up and being overweight.[72] You can't do anything about your genetic make-up, so the best way to raise your HDL cholesterol is to lose weight!

You can also raise your HDL cholesterol level modestly by exercise and regular physical activity.[73] Quitting smoking will also raise your HDL cholesterol level.[74]

Some studies have suggested that saturated fat may also cause colon, prostate, and breast cancer. The truth is we really don't know. Still, it's possible that when you cut out saturated fat to cut your risk of heart disease and lose weight, you might be cutting your risk of colon, prostate, and breast cancer as well.[75, 76]

Trans-fats

In the American diet most *trans*-fats are man-made. *Trans*-fats are made by chemically modifying unsaturated fats by hydrogenation. *Trans*-fats occur in foods such as margarine, vegetable shortening, crackers, cookies, cakes, pies, bread, snack foods, and food fried in partially hydrogenated oils such as French fries and potato chips. Some *trans*-fats are not man-made and occur naturally in foods such as meat, milk, butter, and cheese.[77]

As it turns out, *trans*-fats raise LDL cholesterol levels[78] and contribute to athero-sclerosis and its sequelae, heart disease and stroke.[79,80,81,82] One should avoid eating *trans*-fats whenever possible.

Usually it's not hard to avoid *trans*-fats. For example, many pies contain *trans*-fats, but there are also pies that do not contain *trans*-fats; many breads contain *trans*-fats, but there are also breads that do not contain *trans*-fats; *etc*. You just have to pay attention to the Nutrition Facts labels.

Starting January 1, 2006, the Food and Drug Administration will require all foods to list the amount of *trans*-fats they contain on the labels.[83]

Unfortunately, if foods have less than 0.5 grams (half a gram) of *trans*-fats, the FDA will allow them to be listed as having 0 (zero) *trans*-fat: these foods with low levels of *trans*-fats will however have a "partially hydrogenated" oil listed in the ingredients.

In fact, a major study of male smokers found that men who ate on average 6.2 grams of *trans*-fats a day had a 40% higher risk of dying from heart disease than men who ate on average 1.3 grams of *trans*-fats a day. So even if you eat food that has *trans*-fats listed as 0 on the label, by eating several portions of different foods with, for example, 0.3 or 0.4 grams of *trans*-fats, it is quite easy to eat an amount of *trans*-fats that will raise your risk of heart disease. Of course, eating foods with much more than 0.5 grams of *trans*-fats will greatly increase your risk of heart disease.

What does the "*trans*" in "*trans*-fats" mean? "*Trans*" is a Latin word meaning "on the other side of". Remember the double bond we talked about in unsaturated fats? If the carbon backbone goes in opposite directions on either side of the double bond, then the fat is a "*trans*" fat. If the carbon backbone goes in the same direction on either side of the double bond, then the fat is a "*cis*" fat. ("*Cis*" means "on this side of" in Latin.) "*Cis*" fats are the healthy fats found in nuts, vegetables, corn oil, olives and the like.

The bottom line: avoid foods containing more than 0.5 grams of *trans*-fats. Foods that say 0 grams of *trans*-fats on the label are better, just realize they may have some *trans*-fats in them. Foods that say 0 grams of *trans*-fats on the label and that do not say "partially hydrogenated" in the ingredients are the best.

Red Meat

You should eat less red meat for several reasons.

First, most cuts of red meat are high in fat and have a high caloric density. These cuts of red meat will cause you to gain weight.

Second, red meat is very high in saturated fat. As we just saw, saturated fat causes heart attacks. So it is not surprising that the more meat you eat, the greater your chance of a fatal heart attack.[84] In fact, men between the ages of 45 and 64 who eat meat daily have 3 times the risk of dying of a heart attack than men who don't eat meat.

Third, eating red meat increases your risk of getting colon cancer.[85, 86]

The less red meat you eat, the better.

Burnt, Grilled, and Barbecued Food

Cooking meat at high temperatures creates chemicals called polycyclic aromatic hydrocarbons (PAH).[87] There is compelling evidence that some PAH cause cancer. Many studies have shown that mice and rats fed PAH develop tumors.[88] In addition, studies in people have shown that eating red meat increases the risk of colon cancer. The more well cooked the red meat, the more carcinogenic PAH generated during cooking. It has been shown that people who eat well-done meat have a greater cancer risk than people who eat less well-done meat. Eating well-done red meat increases the risk of colon cancer 9 fold.[89, 90]

What cooking methods have the highest temperatures and generate the most PAH? Grilling, roasting, and frying.

Drying and smoking foods also generate large amounts of PAH.

PAH also occur in cereals, oils and fats, and on the surface of fruits and vegetables, from environmental contamination.

How can you reduce the amount of PAH you eat?[91, 92, 93]

- Eat lean meat and fish.
- Eat smaller portions of grilled and barbecued food.
- Marinate the meat or poultry before cooking it. Marinating meat reduces the amount of PAH created during cooking.[94, 95] Marinate for 4 hours before cooking. You can buy marinade in the store, or you can prepare your own by mixing brown sugar, cider vinegar, garlic, mustard, lemon juice, and a little olive oil.
- Partially pre-cook the meat in a microwave and drain the fat away.

- Avoid contact of food with flames during barbecuing.
- Use less oil for grilling.
- Cook at a lower temperature. Use medium or low heat.
- Do not let fat that drips down onto an open flame and turns into smoke come back up and coat the food with smoke. You can line your grill with foil and poke holes in the foil so that the fat drips down through the holes. This way, when the fat drips on the flames and turns into smoke, most of the smoke cannot come up and coat the food.
- Broil (in which the heat source is above the food) instead of grilling. This way fat will never come in contact with the flames.
- Place meat further from the heat source.
- Avoid charred, burnt, and blackened meat.
- Wash fruit and vegetables.

Remember, more well-done food does not necessarily have a more intense flavor than less well-done food. (Of course, you should always cook meat and fish enough to kill any contaminating bacteria.)

Preserved Meats and Salted Fish

Foods that have been cured and salted may pose a cancer risk. Preserved meats probably increase the risk of colon and rectal cancer.[96] Salt-preserved foods probably increase the risk of stomach cancer. Salted fish increase the risk of a type of head and neck cancer.

Try to limit the amount of preserved meat (for example, bacon, cold cuts, etc.) and salted fish you eat.

Nitrates are present in many preserved meats (hot dogs, cold cuts, etc.) as well as in the drinking water in some places. There is some concern that nitrates are converted in the body to N-nitroso compounds, which have been shown to cause cancer in experimental animals. However, a number of studies have been done in humans and have failed to demonstrate that nitrates cause cancer.[97,98,99] **My advice: it's alright to eat food containing nitrates in moderation, just don't eat food containing nitrates every day.**

Omega-3 Fatty Acids

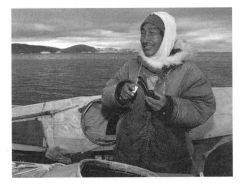

In 1944, towards the end of World War II, Dr. Hugh Sinclair, a young graduate of Oxford, was stationed in northern Canada among the Inuit. Doing eye exams, he observed that the Inuit did not have cholesterol deposits in their retinas that most of the British airmen had. This was sur-

An Inuit hunter

prising, since the Inuit diet consisted mostly of coldwater marine life, name fish, seal, and whale, which are very high in fat.

In 1976 Dr. Sinclair teamed up with two Danish scientists, Dr. Jorn Dyerberg and Dr. Hans Olov Bang, in an expedition by dogsled to North Western Greenland. They found that the Greenland Inuit had very low rates of heart disease despite high fat intakes.[100]

This work was the foundation of research that showed that while some fats—saturated fats—cause heart disease, other fats—omega-3 fatty acids—prevent heart disease.

There are basically 3 different omega-3 fatty acids that people eat. They are called alpha-linolenic acid, EPA*, and DHA†.

Most alpha-linolenic acid in the American diet comes from vegetable oils, especially canola oil and soybean oil. Most EPA and DHA come from fish.

Both the plant-derived omega-3 fatty acids (alpha-linolenic acid) and the marine-derived omega-3 fatty acids (EPA and DHA) reduce the risk of heart disease.[101]

The amount of omega-3 fatty acids in different foods in listed in the tables below.

Realize that fatty fish has more omega-3 fatty acids than lean fish. Yes, fatty fish has a higher caloric density than lean fish, but even fatty fish has a relatively low caloric density and will help you lose weight.

Avoid fried fish, since frying makes process changes the fatty acids in fish. Fried fish are high in unhealthy trans-fats and low in healthy omega-3 fatty acids.

Plant-Derived Omega-3 Fatty Acids

	Alpha-Linolenic Acid Grams/Tablespoon
Canola Oil	1.3
Flaxseed (Linseed) Oil	8.5
Flaxseeds	2.2
Olive Oil	0.1
Soybean Oil	0.9
Walnut Oil	1.4
Walnuts	0.7

Mercury

Thousands of tons of mercury are released into the atmosphere each year both by natural processes, such as volcanic eruptions and erosion of geologic deposits, and man-made pollution, such as burning coal.[102,103] Mercury ends up in the ocean and in freshwater where

*Short for eicosapentaenoic acid.
†Short for docosahexanenoic acid.

Marine-Derived Omega-3 Fatty Acids

	Total Omega-3 (EPA+DHA) in Grams per 6 oz Serving of Fish
Catfish	0.4
Clam	0.5
Cod (Atlantic)	0.3
Cod (Pacific)	0.5
Crab (Alaskan King)	0.7
Flounder and Sole	0.8
Haddock	0.4
Halibut	0.8-2.0
Herring (Atlantic)	3.4
Herring (Pacific)	3.6
Lobster	0.1-0.8
Mackerel	0.7-3.1
Oyster (Eastern)	1.9
Oyster (Farmed)	0.7
Oyster (Pacific)	2.3
Salmon (Atlantic, Farmed)	2.2-3.6
Salmon (Atlantic, Wild)	1.8-3.2
Salmon (Chinook)	3.0
Salmon (Chum)	1.4
Salmon (Pink)	2.2
Salmon (Sockeye)	2.1
Sardines	2.0-3.4
Scallop	0.3
Shrimp	0.5
Trout (Rainbow)	1.7
Tuna (Fresh)	0.5-2.6
Tuna (Light, Canned)	0.5
Tuna (White, Canned)	1.5

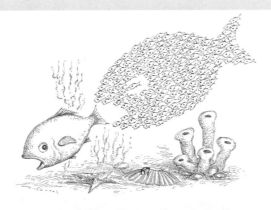

it is concentrated in larger predator fish.[104] In other words, small fish absorb a small amount of mercury from sea- and fresh-water, and the larger fish that eat them—since they eat a large number of the small fish—end up with much more mercury than the small fish, and the very large predator fish that eat the larger fish have even higher levels of mercury.

Mercury poisoning causes neurological disease, which can progress over years.[105]

The FDA recommends that pregnant women, women who may become pregnant, and young children limit their consumption of shark, swordfish, king mackerel, and tilefish.[106] Tuna is not on the FDA list, but it is important to bear in mind that the tuna lobby is large and powerful and has influence over the FDA!

How much mercury-containing fish can one safely eat? This is a complicated question because the studies that have been done have looked only at the easily detectable consequences of poisoning with very high levels of mercury such as severe nerve and brain damage. More subtle neurological effects of low level exposure to mercury, such as slight decreases in intelligence in children and adults, would be very difficult to identify.

One also needs to take into account that fish have many health benefits. Fish have a low caloric density and will help you lose weight. Fish are a particularly good source of *omega*-3 fatty acids,[107] which protect against heart disease, and people who eat fish on a regular basis have a lower risk of dying of heart disease.[108]

Since heart disease is so common and neurological disease from mercury poisoning is so rare, the heart benefits of eating fish outweigh the low risk of neurological disease. That said, since there are so many fish one can choose from, it makes sense to limit your consumption of fish with the very highest amounts of mercury. Pregnant women and children should limit the amount of fish with moderate amounts of mercury they consume as well, since the developing nervous system presumably is more sensitive to mercury toxicity than the adult nervous system.

So what is the take-home advice?

Certain fish contain low levels of mercury.[109,110,111] These include:

Anchovies	Spiny Lobster	Shad
Butterfish	Atlantic Mackerel	Shrimp
Catfish	Chub Mackerel	Smelt
Clams	Mullet	Squid
Cod	Oysters	Tilapia
Crab	Ocean Perch	Freshwater Trout
Crawfish	Pickerel	Tuna—canned, light
Flatfish	Pollock	Whitefish
Haddock	Salmon	Whiting
Hake	Sardines	
Herring	Scallops	

Eat as much of these fish as you want. (Within reason! Don't eat 21 cans of the light, canned tuna a week!)

Certain fish contain moderate levels of mercury. These include:

Bluefish	Monkfish	Skate
Carp	Orange Roughy	Snapper
Grouper	Perch—freshwater	Tilefish—Atlantic
Halibut	Rockfish	Tuna—canned, alba-
American Lobster	Sable	core
Northern Lobster	Sea Bass	Tuna—filet, steak, or
Spanish Mackerel	Striped Bass	sushi
Marlin	Sheepshead	

These fish can probably be eaten by most people without concern for neurological damage. Pregnant women and women who may become pregnant, nursing mothers, and young children should limit the amount of these fish they eat.

Large predator fish that contain higher levels of mercury:

Shark	King Mackerel
Swordfish	Tilefish—Gulf of
	Mexico

You should limit the amount of these fish that you eat. **Certainly pregnant women and women who may become pregnant, nursing mothers, and young children should not eat these fish.**

PCBs in Farmed Salmon

PCBs (polychlorinated biphenyls) are man-made chemicals that were used as insulators in *transformers*, capacitors, and other electrical equipment. Production of PCBs in the U.S. was halted in 1977 because of experimental evidence that PCBs cause cancer in animals.[112] Despite the ban, PCBs produced prior to 1977 remain in the environment and are even detectable in human blood and tissues. PCBs have not been convincingly demonstrated to cause disease in humans.[113] One would expect that if anyone were to get cancer from exposure to PCBs, it would be industrial workers who were exposed to much higher levels of PCBs than people normally are. However, studies of industrial workers exposed to high levels of PCBs showed that they do not have an abnormally high cancer rate.[114] Studies have shown that the children of women who ate salmon from the Great Lakes have cognitive deficits.[115] A few scientists blame contamination of salmon by PCBs. However, there is little reason to suspect that PCBs are the culprit since there are many other chemical contaminants in the Great Lakes. Recently it has been demonstrated that the level of PCBs in farm-raised salmon is 8 times higher than in wild salmon.[116] Whether this makes farm-raised salmon unsafe is debated in the scientific community. My belief is that farm-raised salmon is safe and healthy to eat, since there is no evidence that eating farm-raised salmon causes disease in people. It is probably not such a good idea, though, to eat Great Lakes salmon.

As we just saw, fish such as salmon have many definite real health benefits. There really is no good evidence that there is anything unhealthy about farmed salmon. This is not to say that one should not keep an open mind should studies done in the future show there is something unhealthy about farmed fish—but until then it is not correct to say there is something wrong with farmed fish. Not everyone can afford wild salmon, and it would be a tragedy if people denied themselves the tremendous health benefits of salmon because of media hype about PCBs. You should eat farmed salmon without worry—save your worry for foods that definitely cause disease, such as red meat.

Fiber

Fiber is plant matter that resists digestion by the digestive enzymes in the human digestive system (the mouth, esophagus, stomach, intestines, rectum, and anus).[117] Dietary fiber is composed of plant cell walls, which give plants their rigidity.

Electron micrograph of a potato cell (magnification X 260 at 35mm size). Note the thick cell wall—this is what fiber is made of. The ovoid structures are starch granules.

There are 2 ways to classify fiber.

The first way to classify fiber is by the plant that the fiber comes from. Edible plants fall into 4 categories: fruits, vegetables, cereals (which are grasses that grain is made from), and legumes. Thus, different types of fiber are fruit fiber, vegetable fiber, cereal fiber, and legume fiber.

The second way to classify fiber is by whether it dissolves in water. Soluble fiber is fiber that dissolves in water. Insoluble fiber is fiber that does not dissolve in water.

Eating soluble fiber lowers your LDL cholesterol level about 10%.[118] Several large, controlled clinical trials have demonstrated that a high fiber diet reduces your risk of heart disease about 15%.[119,120]

Scientists believe this is in part because soluble fiber absorbs cholesterol in the intestines, causing it to be excreted in the stool and preventing it from being reabsorbed into the circulation.[121] Whether soluble fiber prevents heart disease only by lowering the LDL cholesterol level or whether there are additional heart-protective properties of soluble fiber is not known.

Healthy foods with the highest amounts of soluble fiber (more than 0.75 grams per 100 grams eaten) include:[122]

Oatmeal	Beans
Avocados	Green Beans
Nectarines	Broccoli
Oranges	Carrots
Peaches	Lima Beans
Pears	Peas
Plums	Potatoes
Prunes	Spinach

Other healthy foods with high amounts of soluble fiber (0.25–0.75 grams per 100 grams eaten) include:

Brown Rice	Chick Peas
Spaghetti	Cabbage
Apples	Cauliflower
Bananas	Onions
Mangos	Green Peppers

The bottom line: **you should eat at least 14 grams of total fiber a day for every 1000 calories you eat.**[123] **So, for example, if you eat 2000 calories a day, this means you should have at least 28 grams of *total* fiber.** This does not mean you should try to eat 28 grams of *soluble* fiber a day, which would be nearly impossible to do! It means that if you are eating 14 grams of total fiber (which includes both soluble fiber and insoluble fiber), you are probably eating enough soluble fiber to have a significant heart protective effect.

Be aware that many commercially available breakfast cereals—while good sources of fiber—have added *trans*-fats and are not heart-healthy. Also, cereal has a relatively high caloric density and will tend to make you gain weight. So eat the healthy cereals listed in the tables in this book—just don't eat a huge portion or you will gain weight.

Fruit, of course, has a low caloric density, so eating fruit will help you lose weight, lower your LDL cholesterol level, and reduce your risk of heart disease![124,125]

Dietary fiber definitely reduces your risk of heart disease. Does dietary fiber also reduce your risk of certain cancers? The answer is far from clear.

A well-designed study of over 500,000 people found that people who ate a large amount of fiber had a decreased risk of cancer of the colon and rectum, and the scientists estimated that doubling the amount of fiber you eat decreases your risk of cancer of the colon and rectum by 40%.[126] In addition, another well-designed study of over 30,000 people found 27% fewer colon adenomas—an early stage of colon cancer—in people who ate a large amount of fiber compared with people who ate a small amount of fiber.[127]

On the other hand, a study of over 40,000 male health professionals[128] and a study of over 80,000 female nurses[129] both found no decreased risk of cancer of the colon and rectum in people who ate a large amount of fiber.

How do we reconcile these contradictory results? I am not certain, but one possibility may relate to the way the different studies take into account factors other than fiber. In other words, people who eat more fiber tend to eat less red meat and more fruits and vegetables. Eating red meat—irrespective of the amount of fiber you eat—increases your risk of cancer of the colon and rectum.[130,131,132] Fruits and vegetables may contain compounds other than fiber that protect against cancer of the colon and rectum, although this is not certain.[133,134,135] So it may be that eating less red meat and eating more fruits and vegetables, rather than eating more fiber *per se*, reduces your risk of cancer of the colon and rectum. It may be that the studies that found no benefit to fiber took into account these other factors better than the studies that found benefit to fiber.

What is the bottom line? To avoid cancer of the colon and rectum, eat less red meat. Eat more fiber to lower your LDL cholesterol level and your risk of heart disease. Whether or not eating more fiber reduces your risk of cancer of the colon and rectum is not known.

Eating more fiber has other beneficial effects.

Even after adjusting for BMI*, people who consume a large amount of cereal fiber have been found to have about a 30% lower chance of developing type 2 diabetes (the more common type of diabetes in adults) than people who consume a small amount of cereal fiber.[136,137,138] (A large amount of cereal fiber is more than 8 grams of cereal fiber a day, and a small amount of cereal fiber is less than 3 grams of cereal fiber a day.) Interestingly, eating a large amount of fruit fiber or vegetable fiber neither decreases nor increases the likelihood of getting diabetes.

---

*It was important to adjust for BMI since the heavier someone is, the greater their risk for diabetes. In other words, for people who are equally overweight, the risk of developing type 2 diabetes is 30% lower in those who consume a large amount of cereal fiber than in those who consume a small amount of cereal fiber.

Eating more insoluble fiber, when taken with a sufficient amount of water or other liquids, reduces constipation.[139] Insoluble fiber, when taken with sufficient liquids, can help prevent hemorrhoids and can sometimes cure hemorrhoids.[140] Eating more insoluble fiber will also reduce your risk of an infectious process of the colon called diverticulitis and of a disease of massive bleeding from the colon called bleeding diverticulosis.[141,142]

Whole Grains

Grains are the fruits of grasses.[143] In the United States, the grain products that we eat the most of are wheat (by far the leader), corn, and rice products.[144] We eat lesser amounts of oat, rye, and barley products.

Each grain consists of concentric layers.[145] From outermost to innermost the layers of a grain are: the husk, which protects the plant embryo and is hard and inedible; the bran, which is the fruit wall and protects the embryo, provides nutrients for the growing plant seedling, and provides biological signals that guide the development of the seedling; the germ, which is the grain plant embryo; and the endosperm, which provides nutrients for the growing seedling.

For wheat, the bran and the germ represent only 17% of the weight of the edible portion of the wheat grain but contain 80% of the fiber. There are very few calories in the bran and the germ. The germ contains polyunsaturated fatty acids. There are many plant chemicals (also called phytochemicals) in the bran and the germ.

In contrast, the endosperm consists mostly of starch and is low in fiber and relatively high in calories.

A "whole grain" food contains all the edible parts of the grain: the bran, the germ, and the endosperm.[146]

Examples of whole grain foods that Americans eat include whole grain breads, some breakfast cereals, whole grain pasta, oatmeal, and brown rice.

Originally all grains were whole grains. Grain refining as we know it today was developed in the 1880s with the introduction of steel rollers to mill grain by companies such as General Mills.

Refined grain contains only the endosperm. The bran and the germ are removed.

Examples of refined grain foods include white bread, bagels, rolls, pastries, some breakfast cereals, white and durum flour pasta, and white rice.

"Whole grain" does not mean that the grain in a food is intact—it just means that food contains all 3 layers of the grain. Most grain products eaten today—whether whole grain or refined grain—are made from flour, which is made by grinding up the grain. The difference is that whole grain flour is made simply by grinding up the grain, while refined grain flour is made by grinding up the grain and then removing the germ and the bran. So almost all whole grain foods we eat are made from ground up grain and contain ground up endosperm, ground up germ, and ground up bran. Refined grain foods are made from ground up endosperm only.

People who eat 2–3 servings of whole grain foods have a 20–30% lower risk of heart disease than people who eat little whole grain foods.[147,148,149] How much is 1 serving of whole grain food? 1 slice of dark bread; 1 cup of cold breakfast cereal, brown rice, or cooked oatmeal; or 1 tablespoon of wheat bran.

The part of the whole grain that appears to reduce the risk of heart disease is the bran: a well-designed study found that men who consume a large amount of added bran have a 30% lower risk of heart disease than men who ate no added bran. (Men who ate added germ had the same risk of heart disease as men who ate no added germ.)

Interestingly, while the fiber in whole grains certainly is part of the reason why whole grain foods lead to a lower risk of heart disease, the research indicates that there is something in the whole grain foods other than the fiber that is responsible for part of the heart-protecting effect.

People who eat a large amount of whole grain foods have been found to have a 30–40% lower risk of developing type 2 diabetes (even after adjusting for BMI).[150,151] It is unclear if this effect is wholly due to the cereal fiber in whole grain foods or if there are other substances in whole grain foods that protect against diabetes.

The bottom line: eat whole grain foods: they lower your risk of heart disease and diabetes. You get the greatest benefits from eating 2–3 servings a day.

Fruits and Vegetables

Fruits and vegetables are healthy for several reasons.

First, fruits and vegetables have a very low caloric density, and so will help you lose weight (as long as you don't eat a very large amount!)

Second, fruits and vegetables are believed to improve your blood cholesterol levels and reduce your risks of heart disease and stroke.[152] People who eat fruits and vegetables 3 or more times a day have about a 25% lower risk of heart disease than people who eat fruits and vegetables less than once a day.[153]

Third, eating fruits and vegetables may reduce your chances of getting cancer, although we don't know for sure.[154,155] Eating fruits and vegetables probably reduces your risk of getting cancer of the oral cavity, esophagus, stomach, colon, or rectum. Plant foods contain a number of ingredients, including micronutrients, polyunsaturated fatty acids, and natural compounds called glucosinolates and flavonoids, that may stop cancer cells from dividing and may kill cancer cells.[156] The evidence for this is far from clear however.

Fourth, eating fruits and certain vegetables will reduce your risk for certain eye diseases. People who eat 3 or more servings of fruit a day have been found to have a 36% lower risk of macular degeneration than people who eat less than 1½ servings of fruit a day.[157] Eating vegetables might also reduce your risk of macular degeneration.[158] Spinach and broccoli contain a molecule called lutein, and men over 45 who consume a large amount of lutein have been found to have a 19% lower risk of forming cataracts.[159] It is possible that lutein, which is an anti-oxidant, soaks up oxygen free radicals that cause cataracts.

How much fruit and vegetables should you eat a day? Eight servings appears to be the amount that provides the greatest protection against disease.[160,161] This includes fruits, berries, and vegetables as well as jams, nectars, and juices.* If you don't want to eat eight servings a day, well, 4 servings is better than 2 servings.

Nuts

Eating nuts dramatically reduces the risk of heart disease. This has been conclusively proven by several well-designed large epidemiologic studies. [157,158] People who ate more than 5 ounces of nuts (including peanuts) a week had about a 35% lower chance of heart disease.

The reason for this beneficial effect is not known but may relate to the high amounts of monounsaturated fats in nuts.

The same degree of beneficial effect of nuts and peanuts was not seen for peanut butter. Perhaps this is because most commercially bought peanut butter has added hydrogenated fat. When you go to the grocery store, be sure to buy "natural" peanut butter, which does not contain harmful additives such as hydrogenated fat. Though this has not been proven, it is extremely likely that natural peanut butter lowers the risk of heart disease as much as nuts and peanuts do.

The one catch about nuts is that nuts have a very high caloric density, and eating a large amount of nuts could cause you to gain weight. My advice would be to eat between 5 and 10 ounces of nuts a week once you have achieved your goal weight. Because nuts have such a high caloric density, it makes sense not to eat nuts until you achieve your goal weight. For those people who find themselves unable to lose weight for psychological reasons (e.g. binge eaters), my advice is to eat 5 ounces of nuts a week to get the heart benefit and to cut calories somewhere else.

How much is one ounce of nuts? 24 almonds, 6–8 Brazil nuts, 18 cashews, 12 hazelnuts, 10–12 macadamia nuts, 28 peanuts, 20 pecan halves, 47 pistachio nuts, or 14 walnut halves.

Salt

You do need to consume some salt (sodium chloride). There is sodium in every cell in your body, and sodium is involved in every biologic process. If you consume too little sodium, you will rapidly become dehydrated. In the conditions our ancestors faced, enough sodium was not always readily available. Perhaps this is why our sense of taste is designed such that people like salty foods so much.

---

*Do jams, nectars, and juices have the same beneficial effects as whole fruits and vegetables? Perhaps, perhaps not. We simply do not know yet.

For many years it has been dogma in the medical community that consuming too much salt causes high blood pressure. It is well established that high blood pressure causes cardiovascular disease including stroke. So it was believed that reducing salt consumption could reduce the risk of cardiovascular disease.

Much of this dogma stems from studies on rodents done in the 1950s and 1960s under conditions that do not at all mimic those of human populations.[164] In 1960, Dr. Lewis Dahl of the Brookhaven National Laboratory published a famous graph comparing sodium intake in different groups of people with rates of high blood pressure. This graph was reproduced in many medical textbooks and became a cornerstone of the belief in the medical community that sodium consumption causes high blood pressure. But Dr. Dahl did not publish how he acquired this data. He appears to have created it out of thin air!

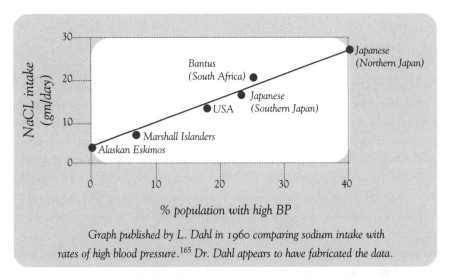

Graph published by L. Dahl in 1960 comparing sodium intake with rates of high blood pressure.[165] Dr. Dahl appears to have fabricated the data.

This was followed by a series of flawed, uncontrolled human studies conducted by several groups in the late 1960s and early 1970s that erroneously reported that decreasing sodium intake dramatically decreases blood pressure. This led to the 1979 Surgeon General's report that asserted that sodium intake was a major cause of high blood pressure.[166]

Having been established as dogma endorsed by the government, accepted by the medical community, and widely believed by the public at large, the idea that salt causes high blood pressure led to several popular myths. Among these myths are the beliefs that salt consumption has increased dramatically in the last century, that humans consume far more sodium than they require, and that normal people would benefit from reducing their sodium consumption. It also led to the myth that the high rates of high blood pressure among African-Americans is due to a greater use of salt.

In fact, the blood pressure of different people responds differently to increases in sodium intake. Increasing sodium intake causes the blood pressure of some people to rise but does not have this effect on other people.[167] There are even some people whose blood pressure decreases with increased sodium intake.

Finally, between 1984 and 1988, a large, well-designed study of 10,000 people in 32 countries was conducted.[168] This study did not find that populations with higher sodium intakes had higher rates of high blood pressure.

This study did find an association between higher sodium intakes and a faster rise of blood pressure with age. However, independent statistical analysis of the data concluded that it would be incorrect to draw the conclusion that decreasing sodium intake in normal individuals would slow the rise of blood pressure with age.

Several well-designed large-scale statistical analyses of blood pressure and sodium intake were conducted in the 1990s. These studies found that reducing sodium in the diet of normal individuals by 30-50% decreased the systolic blood pressure by only 1-2 points and decreased the diastolic blood pressure by 0-1 points.[169,170,171]

A recent study even found that people with lower sodium intakes had a higher risk of cardiovascular disease and mortality.[172] In fact, there have now been multiple studies that have found no benefit to a low sodium diet in terms of reducing the risk of cardiovascular disease in healthy people.

The relationship between nutrient consumption and blood pressure appears to be complicated. People with a low calcium intake (less than 400 mg daily for men and less than 800 mg daily for women) appear to increase their blood pressure with increased sodium intake, but people with normal calcium intakes do not appear to increase their blood pressure with increased sodium intakes.[173]

While decreasing sodium intake barely decreases blood pressure in most people without high blood pressure, it should be noted that some people have "salt-sensitive hypertension": that is, the more sodium they consume, the higher their blood pressure. People with salt-sensitive high blood pressure increase their average blood pressure more than 5% when they are eating a high sodium diet. About 50% of people with high blood pressure have salt-sensitive high blood pressure.[174] So if you have high blood pressure, you should discuss it with your doctor and consider a trial of a low sodium diet. If your blood pressure falls with the low sodium diet, you have salt-sensitive high blood pressure and should limit the amount of sodium you consume. But if your blood pressure does not fall with a low sodium diet, you may have salt-resistant high blood pressure, and there is no point for you to make great efforts to avoid sodium.

If decreasing sodium intake is not the answer to lowering blood pressure, what is? The best answer to date comes from the DASH* study.[175] The DASH study evaluated the effects of a diet high in fruits, vegetables, and low fat dairy products. The DASH study found that for people without high blood pressure (systolic pressure less than 140 and diastolic pressure less than 90[†]), eating such a diet reduced the systolic pressure by 4 points and the diastolic pressure by 2 points. The DASH study also found that for people with high blood pressure (either systolic pressure greater than 140 or diastolic pressure greater than 90 or both), eating such a diet reduced the systolic pressure by 11 points and the diastolic pressure by 6 points.

If the relationship between sodium and high blood pressure is unclear, are there any problems associated with a high sodium intake?

High sodium intake has been linked with certain cancers. A high sodium intake is believed to increase the chance of developing head and neck cancer and stomach cancer.[176,177,178] I do wonder though about the extent to which sodium plays a role in the development of these cancers and the extent to which other factors, such as poor refrigeration and infection with the bacterium *Helicobacter pylori*, are important.

The bottom line: to avoid high blood pressure, eat a diet rich in fruits and vegetables with sufficient low fat and nonfat dairy products.

If you do not have high blood pressure, I would not worry too much about sodium intake. It is reasonable to limit the amount of heavily salted food you eat.

If you do have high blood pressure, see your doctor. A diet rich in fruits and vegetables and sufficient low fat and nonfat dairy products is certainly a good idea for you. You may be a "salt-sensitive" individual, and a trial of a low sodium diet is reasonable. If lowering your sodium intake lowers your blood pressure—great!—stick with it. But if lowering your sodium intake does not lower your blood pressure, it may be pointless to continue a low sodium diet. Certainly if you cannot lower your blood pressure with diet and weight loss, you should talk with your doctor about starting medication for high blood pressure in order to decrease your risks for stroke and heart disease.

The Golden Gate Diet allows you to eat both non-salty and salty foods. Some people—"salt-sensitive individuals"—increase their blood pressure when they eat salty foods, whereas other people do not increase their blood pressure when they eat salty foods. If you find that eating more salty foods increases your blood pressure, eat less salty foods.

---

* Dietary Approaches to Stop Hypertension

† Your blood pressure is reported as 2 numbers. The first number is called the systolic pressure, and the second number is called the diastolic pressure. So if your blood pressure is 120/75, your systolic pressure is 120, and your diastolic pressure is 75.

Vitamins and Minerals

It's a good idea to take a vitamin pill every day. It has been known for many years that taking vitamins prevents several diseases, such as scurvy and pellagra.

The first evidence that nutrients in certain foods prevent specific diseases was discovered by Dr. James Lind, a Scottish Naval surgeon. In 1747, Dr. Lind was the surgeon aboard H.M.S. Salisbury, which was patrolling the English channel during the War of Austrian Succession. Of the Salisbury's 350 men, 80 contracted scurvy, a disease with symptoms such as bleeding gums, rotten teeth, and joint pains.

Dr. Lind selected 12 men from the crew and divided them into six pairs. Every day he gave one pair seawater, one pair a mixture of garlic, mustard, and horseradish, one pair vinegar, one pair an elixir which he did not describe, one pair a quart of cider, and one pair two oranges and a lemon. The first four pairs reported no change, the pair given cider had a slight improvement in their symptoms, and the pair given oranges and lemons made a dramatic recovery.[179]

Vitamins are not just important for preventing diseases that are relatively rare these days, such as scurvy. It turns out that vitamin B_{12} and folate are important for preventing vascular disease, such as heart disease.

. While one can certainly get enough vitamins and minerals through a well-balanced diet, an easier and more certain way to get the vitamins and minerals you need is to take one multi-vitamin pill a day. A multi-vitamin pill will supply you with 100% of the RDA (Recommended Daily Allowance) of most vitamins and minerals. Multi-vitamin pills can be found in any drugstore.

It is unnecessary to take more than one vitamin pill, and taking pills of individual vitamins and minerals is a waste of money. There are some exceptions for people with certain medical conditions. For example, if your iron level is low, your doctor might tell you to take an iron pill in addition to the vitamin pill. And if you're not getting enough calcium in your diet, it makes sense to take a calcium pill.)

In general, one should avoid taking large doses of vitamins. Except in a few very unusual circumstances, there is no health benefit to taking large doses of vitamins. In addition, taking much larger than the recommended doses of vitamins can cause health problems. For example, taking high doses of vitamin A can cause liver fibrosis among other problems.[180]

Is it better to get your vitamins and minerals from the foods you eat than from a multi-vitamin pill? To the best of our current knowledge, the answer is no. It makes no difference whether you get the vitamins and minerals from the food you eat or you get the vitamins and minerals from a pill.

Studies have been done where subjects will eat a vitamin pill, and then, after a period of time, the subject's blood will be drawn and the level of the vitamin in the blood tested. These studies have shown that vitamins and minerals in a pill are absorbed by the intestines into the body effectively.[181,182]

U.S. Pharmacopeia (USP), a non-governmental organization advised by scientists, tests multi-vitamin pills to make sure the vitamins and minerals in them dissolve in dilute acid, which simulates conditions in the stomach.[183]

If you do not take a multi-vitamin pill, you run the risk of developing a vitamin deficiency, particularly when you are dieting. It is unnecessary to worry about getting all the different vitamins you need in your food if you take a multi-vitamin pill every day.

Vitamin B_{12} and folate

Vitamin B_{12} and folate are important for preventing vascular disease, such as heart disease. It is possible that vitamin B_{12} and folate may reduce your risk of Alzheimer disease, although this is not certain.

One byproduct of protein break-down is a molecule called homocysteine.[184] High levels of homocysteine are toxic to arteries and veins and can cause atherosclerosis.[185] To date, more than 80 studies have demonstrated that high levels of homocysteine in the blood increase the risk of heart disease, stroke, and peripheral vascular disease.[186]

While the cause of high levels of homocysteine appears to be in part genetic, it can also be caused by deficiency of vitamin B_{12} or folate.[187,188] This is because vitamin B_{12} and folate are important in regenerating homocysteine back into the amino acid methionine, which is a protein "building block".[189]

So if you don't get enough vitamin B_{12} and folate, you are at risk for heart disease, stroke, and peripheral vascular disease.[190]

Healthy sources of vitamin B_{12} include nonfat dairy products, fish, and some breakfast cereals, and healthy sources of folate include fruits, peas, beans, and leafy green vegetables such as spinach.

Alzheimer's disease is a disorder of progressive brain dysfunction. Alzheimer's disease destroys a person's memory and abilities to learn and reason, to communicate, and to perform the basic tasks of daily life.

Can changing your diet reduce your risk for Alzheimer's disease?

The truth is that no one really knows, but there is some evidence that making some changes to your diet might reduce your risk of Alzheimer's disease.

Some studies point to a possible role for homocysteine in Alzheimer's disease. These studies have found that people with high blood levels of homocysteine are at increased risk for Alzheimer's disease.[191] In addition, some studies suggest that people with deficiencies of folate and of vitamin B_{12} have elevated blood levels of homocysteine and have higher rates of Alzheimer's disease.[192,193]

Unfortunately, other studies have found no relationship between high blood levels of homocysteine and Alzheimer's disease.[194,195]

There may be dietary risk factors for Alzheimer's disease other than vitamin B_{12} and folate. Certain people, because of their genetic make-up, are at higher risk for Alzheimer's disease. People with a common gene variant are at much higher risk of getting Alzheimer's disease.[196] A recent study found that among people with this inherited gene variant, those who consumed a large number of calories and a large amount of fat had twice the risk of getting Alzheimer's disease that people with the same gene variant who did not consume a large number of calories and a large amount of fat had.[197] But for people who did not have the gene variant, it made no difference how many calories and how much fat they consumed.

The bottom line: make sure you get enough vitamin B_{12} and folate to reduce your risks of heart disease, stroke, and peripheral vascular disease. Healthy sources of vitamin B_{12} include nonfat dairy products, fish, and some breakfast cereals, and healthy sources of folate include fruits, peas, beans, and leafy green vegetables such as spinach. You can also get enough vitamin B_{12} and folate by taking a vitamin pill.

Unfortunately, there is no conclusive evidence that changing your diet will decrease your risk of Alzheimer's disease. However, you *might* decrease your risk of Alzheimer's disease if you eat healthy foods high in folate and vitamin B_{12}, if you take a vitamin pill every day, or if you choose a diet low in calories. Again, while the evidence is not strong, I would certainly do this if Alzheimer disease runs in your family.

Anti-oxidants with emphasis on vitamin E, vitamin C, and coenzyme Q_{10}

A by-product of many reactions in the body—particularly reactions of the immune system—is a molecule called the oxygen free radical.*

Oxygen free radicals can react with DNA in the cells, damaging the DNA. This damaged DNA could cause cancer.

An anti-oxidant is a molecule that absorbs oxygen free radicals. Because they can "soak up" oxygen free radicals, scientists believe anti-oxidants prevent oxygen free radi-

---

* What is an oxygen free radical? It is an oxygen molecule with an unpaired electron. The unpaired electron is extremely unstable and reactive—which is why the oxygen free radical damages cellular components such as DNA.

cals from damaging DNA. And because anti-oxidants prevent DNA damage, some scientists believe anti-oxidants could prevent cancer.

As you may recall, one of the particles that *transports* cholesterol and fats in the bloodstream is LDL (low density lipoprotein). Oxygen free radicals can react with fats in LDL, creating oxidized LDL. One theory is that atherosclerosis—the process underlying most heart disease—is started by oxidized LDL.

Again, because they can "soak up" oxygen free radicals, some scientists believe anti-oxidants could prevent the creation of oxidized LDL. And because anti-oxidants prevent the creation of oxidized LDL, it is believed anti-oxidants could prevent atherosclerosis and heart disease.

So the theory has been that anti-oxidants prevent cancer and that anti-oxidants prevent heart disease. The popular press has been quick to jump on the anti-oxidant bandwagon. Perhaps as a result, possibly as many as 30% of Americans are taking an anti-oxidant supplement. But is it true? Do anti-oxidants really prevent cancer and heart disease?

The three anti-oxidant molecules that have garnered the most attention both in the popular press and among the scientific community are: vitamin E, vitamin C, and coenzyme Q10.

In most nutrition stores you can purchase natural vitamin E, which is derived from food sources, or synthetic vitamin E, which is derived from non-food sources. Vitamin E is a mixture of chemicals, and in humans the most common form of vitamin E is called *alpha*-tocopherol.

Vitamin E has been shown to have anti-oxidant activity: that is, it can "soak up" oxygen free radicals. For this reason vitamin E has been touted as a cancer-preventing and heart disease-preventing compound.

However, no studies in humans have ever shown convincingly that vitamin E prevents cancer.[198] The results of studies of the effects of vitamin E on heart disease are mixed.

Of 32 animal studies of atherosclerosis that compared animals fed food with high doses of vitamin E with animals fed normal food, 9 studies found a beneficial effect of high dose vitamin E, 19 studies found no effect of high dose vitamin E, and 4 studies found a harmful effect of high dose vitamin E.[199] In contrast, 4 of 5 studies that compared *vitamin E-supplemented diets* with *vitamin E-deficient diets* found beneficial effects of vitamin E.

Human studies have been disappointing. Five different large studies of vitamin E failed to find a convincing benefit of vitamin E.[200,201,202,203,304] Only two of these studies even hinted at the possibility of vitamin E having a role in preventing heart disease. A recent analysis found that in 9 of 11 studies, the risk of dying was increased in people who took a vitamin E supplement.[205] This analysis suggested you should avoid taking 400 IU or more of vitamin E a day. It should be said though that this analysis had limitations.

In fact, evidence suggests that vitamin E can have pro-oxidant effects:* that is, that vitamin E can accelerate the rate of formation of oxidized LDL.[206,207]

If all this weren't complicated enough, it turns out that vitamin E has numerous other effects in the body that have nothing to do with it being an anti-oxidant.[208]

It is not clear that taking a vitamin E pill will prevent heart disease. Taking a vitamin E pill might increase your risk of dying. At this time, I do not recommend taking a vitamin E pill. I think it is reasonable to get normal amount of vitamin E in the diet—and you can get a normal amount of vitamin E from foods such as nuts, oils, and vegetables.

Several studies in which patients with advanced cancer were given supplemental vitamin C have not shown any decrease in the death rate.[209] There is no evidence that taking vitamin C prevents cancer or heart disease. Of course, the recommended daily dosage of vitamin C is necessary to prevent scurvy, but you don't need to take a separate vitamin C pill to prevent scurvy. There is enough vitamin C in a standard multi-vitamin pill.

Since there is no evidence that taking a vitamin C pill prevents heart disease or cancer, I do not recommend taking a vitamin C pill. Of course, you should get the normal daily dose of vitamin C to prevent scurvy—you can do this by taking a standard multi-vitamin pill or by eating foods containing vitamin C.

There have been no controlled trials to investigate whether coenzyme Q_{10} can prevent or cure cancer or heart disease, so there is simply no evidence that coenzyme Q_{10} prevents or cures cancer or heart disease.

Since there is no good evidence that taking a coenzyme Q_{10} pill is beneficial, I do not recommend taking a coenzyme Q_{10} pill.

There are of course other anti-oxidants. The truth is that there are no good studies that demonstrate that taking anti-oxidant pills is of health benefit.

The bottom line: I do not recommend taking anti-oxidant supplements. The scientific evidence to date suggests that taking pills containing anti-oxidants does not reduce your risks of cancer or heart disease.

Calcium and Vitamin D

Calcium plays a role in many different processes in the body. Calcium phosphate is by far the most common mineral in bone. Calcium makes bones strong.

In the disease osteoporosis, bones lose calcium over time. The bones thus become weak and fracture easily.

Adequate calcium intake is important to help prevent osteoporosis.[210] This is particularly true for women, who are at higher risk for osteoporosis.

---

* Why would some studies suggest alpha-tocopherol is an anti-oxidant yet other studies suggest alpha-tocopherol is a pro-oxidant? It may have to do with the strength of the oxidizing source. In the test tube a very strong oxidizing source can be added, so that a large number of oxygen free radicals are generated. These oxygen free radicals can react with alpha-tocopherol to create modified alpha-tocopherol that itself has a free radical. Multiple molecules of radicalized alpha-tocopherol can then react with each other, neutralizing each other. However, in the human body, a relatively small number of oxygen free radicals may be present, generating only a few molecules of radicalized alpha-tocopherol. These few molecules of radicalized alpha-tocopherol may not be able to find each other, since they are few in number, and so would be unable to neutralize each other. Radicalized alpha-tocopherol appears to be more effective at entering the LDL particle than oxygen free radicals, so alpha-tocopherol could transport free radicals within LDL, accelerating the formation of oxidized LDL.

Vitamin D plays important roles in maintaining normal bone calcium levels.[211]

Vitamin D increases absorption of calcium and phosphate by the intestine. Vitamin D also stimulates the kidney to absorb calcium, preventing calcium from being passed out into the urine. These actions of vitamin D keep calcium and phosphate in the body, so they can be added to the bones.

The actions of vitamin D on bones and on certain glands in the neck called the parathyroid glands are complicated. Suffice it to say that vitamin D acts to maintain strong, healthy bones.

Your skin makes vitamin D when it is exposed to sunlight. Many people who live in Northern climates don't get much sun, and in this case vitamin D can be obtained in the diet. Large amounts of vitamin D occur naturally in only a few types of foods—fish, egg yolk, and liver. Of these, only fish is healthy, since egg yolk and liver are high in saturated fats. However, in the United States vitamin D is added to some foods—milk in particular. Skim milk is a good source of vitamin D.

In addition to calcium, consuming an adequate amount of vitamin D is helpful in preventing osteoporosis.[212]

The addition of vitamin D to milk has been an important public health measure. While we know now that adding vitamin D to milk is important in preventing osteoporosis in older Americans, orig-

inally vitamin D was added to milk because of the disease rickets. Rickets is a disease that develops in children who both don't get adequate sun exposure and don't get vitamin D in the diet. Children with rickets develop bowlegs, long bone deformities, and dwarfism.[213] At the turn of the 20th century, the vast majority of children in the cities of England and the United States had rickets.[214] After the routine addition of vitamin D to milk in the 1940s, rickets was practically abolished. Rare cases of rickets still do occur in the United States in dark-skinned infants, and it is important that pregnant women and children consume an adequate amount of vitamin D.[215]

Consuming adequate calcium is impor-

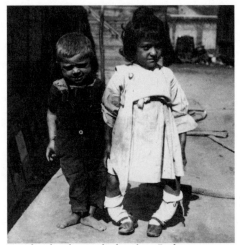

A girl with rickets and a boy from Budapest, Hungary, 1895.

tant for several other reasons in addition to maintaining strong bones. Adequate calcium intake is helpful in controlling high blood pressure and has a beneficial effect on the blood cholesterol level.[216] Adequate calcium intake may reduce the risk of colon cancer.[217]

The National Academy of Sciences recommends that adults under 50 consume 1000 mg of calcium a day and that adults over 50 consume 1200 mg of calcium a day.[218] They recommend children between the ages of 9 and 18—whose bones are growing—consume 1300 mg of calcium a day.

It is probably not necessary to consume as much calcium as recommended by the National Academy of Sciences. These guidelines were based on studies in which patients increased their consumption of *both* calcium and vitamin D. The vitamin D, rather than the calcium, was probably the important change. Recently, several excellent longitudinal studies have found no decrease in fractures in women who were consuming high amounts of calcium.[219,220]

My advice: consume at least 800 mg a day of calcium. Children aged 9 and older and adolescents may benefit from consuming more calcium than this. Understand that there may be no benefit to consuming 800 mg a day as opposed to 400 mg a day, but until further research is done this is a safe, reasonable approach. **Take a multi-vitamin pill to ensure that you are consuming an adequate amount of vitamin D.**

Men should probably avoid very high intakes of calcium (greater than 2000 mg a day), since high calcium intakes appear to increase the risk of prostate cancer.[221,222]

An 8 ounce glass of skim milk contains about 300 mg of calcium. One cup of low fat yogurt contains 415 mg of calcium.

Healthy Foods with a High Amount of Calcium[223]

		Calcium (mg)
Low fat yogurt	8 oz	415
Orange juice with added calcium	8 oz	350
Canned sardines (includes bones)	3 oz	325
Skim milk	8 oz	302
Spinach	1 cup	245
Raisin bran cereal	1 cup	238
Collards	1 cup	226
Turnip greens	1 cup	197
Soup made with skim milk	1 cup	186
Canned salmon (includes bones)	3 oz	181
Pudding made with skim milk	4 oz	153
Nonfat cheese	1 slice	145
Tofu	1 piece 2 ½"x2 ¾"x1"	133

Note that some foods high in calcium are high in fat and calories. Often nonfat equivalents are available (for example, skim milk, nonfat yogurt).

People who are dieting may have difficulty consuming 800 mg of calcium a day. Of course, I recommend everyone take a multi-vitamin pill daily, although multi-vitamin pills have a relatively small amount of calcium—between 100 and 200 mg. If you are having difficulty meeting the daily calcium recommendation, my advice would be to take a calcium supplement pill. Most calcium supplement pills contain between 500 and 600 mg of calcium.

People who are taking medications should discuss taking a calcium pill with their doctor before starting the calcium, since calcium can interfere with certain medications.

Is it worse to take calcium from a pill than to get it from foods? No! Several studies suggest that calcium from a pill is absorbed just as well as calcium from milk.[224,225] It is best to take a calcium pill that contains vitamin D. You should take the calcium pill during mealtime, since more calcium is absorbed when it is eaten with food.[226]

Iron

Iron is the mineral in blood that carries oxygen throughout the body. Sufficient iron intake is important to prevent a low blood count. This is particularly true for young children, teenage girls, and women of child-bearing age. Listed below are some foods with a high amount of iron:[227]

Shellfish such as shrimp, clams, mussels, and oysters
Ready-to-eat cereals with added iron
Turkey dark meat (but remove skin to reduce fat!)
Sardines
Spinach
Cooked dry beans, peas, and lentils
Enriched and whole-grain breads

Yogurt

Yogurt may be a particularly good food for many women. A common infection of the female genital tract is fungal vaginitis (yeast infection). It has been reported that eating yogurt may decrease the risk of fungal vaginitis in women with a history of fungal vaginitis.[228] Unfortunately, there have been no large, well-controlled studies to examine potential benefits of eating yogurt for decreasing the risk of vaginitis.

Why might yogurt decrease the infection risk? Often yogurt contains live cultures of the bacterium *Lactobacillus acidophilus*. Ingested *Lactobacillus* can colonize the vagina and may produce antifungal compounds.

While we do not know for certain that yogurt can prevent vaginal infection, it is good to know that it may have this benefit.

My advice: women with vaginal infection should go to their doctors for evaluation. This is important to make sure there is not a more serious problem causing the vaginal infection.

If the infection is found to be a simple fungal infection, once the infection is controlled with antifungal medication, eating yogurt may prevent the infection from coming back.

How much yogurt? 8 ounces a day.

Of course, it would make sense to eat yogurt with active (live) cultures of *Lactobacillus*, since presumably dead *Lactobacillus* would not be able to colonize the vagina. To tell if a particular brand of yogurt contains active cultures of *Lactobacillus*, check the ingredients. I would also recommend you choose nonfat (or perhaps 1% fat) yogurt to avoid eating saturated fat.

Artificial Sweeteners: Saccharin (Sweet'N Low®), Aspartame (NutraSweet®, Equal®), and Sucralose (Splenda®)

People like to eat sweet food. The problem is that sugar has a lot of calories. Artificial sweeteners make food sweet but give you zero or near-zero calories.

The three most commonly used artificial sweeteners are saccharin, which goes by the brand name Sweet'N Low®; aspartame, which goes by the brand names NutraSweet® and Equal®; and sucralose, which goes by the brand name Splenda®.

Saccharin is made by chemically modifying the compound toluene. Saccharin is 300 times sweeter than sugar.

Saccharin causes bladder cancer in male rats when the rats are fed high levels of saccharin.[229] Saccharin causes the formation of solid matter in the male rat bladder that is toxic to the bladder.[230] The male rat appears to be far more susceptible to formation of this toxic solid matter than humans are because rat urine is much more highly concentrated than human urine and contains high levels of protein that are not present in human urine.[231] Studies of humans have not found any link between saccharin and cancer. One should bear in mind that people live a lot longer than rats and that subtle cancer-causing effects of long-term consumption of saccharin might not show up in human studies. My own feeling is that it is very likely that saccharin is safe to eat.

Saccharin has a long shelf life and is frequently used in fountain sodas for this reason. Saccharin is not destroyed by high temperatures and can be used in baking.

Aspartame is made by joining two amino acids, aspartic acid and phenylalanine. (Amino acids are the "building blocks" of proteins.) Aspartame is 180 times sweeter than sugar.

Many human and animals studies of the safety of aspartame have been done. No link between aspartame and cancer has been found, and in fact, aspartame has not been found to cause any health problems for the general population.[232] Aspartame has been on the market since 1981, long enough one would presume for long-term effects to become evident.

People with the genetic disease phenylketonuria need to limit their intake of the amino acid phenylalanine and should not consume aspartame.

Aspartame is destroyed by high temperatures: for this reason it is not a common choice for use in baked goods.

Sucralose is made by chemically modifying sugar with chlorine atoms. Sucralose is 600 times sweeter than sugar.

Studies have not found any link between sucralose and cancer, nor have they found any harmful health effects of sucralose.[233] Sucralose has been on the market in the United States since 1998.

Sucralose has a long shelf life, is not destroyed by high temperatures, and can be used in baking.

It seems very likely that all three artificial sweeteners, saccharin, aspartame, and sucralose, are safe to consume. Although there is no evidence that saccharin causes cancer in humans, since saccharin has been shown to cause rat bladder tumors, and since you can just as easily eat aspartame, to me it makes sense to choose aspartame. Sucralose is very likely to be safe to eat, but since sucralose has not been on the market for as long as aspartame, again I would stick with aspartame: if there is a subtle long-term effect of sucralose, it might take time for us to become aware of it. The exception is that since aspartame decomposes when heated, use saccharin or sucralose to sweeten baked goods.

Of course, eating sugar causes you to gain weight, and the health consequences of being overweight are severe! If you are overweight it is far healthier to eat any of the artificial sweeteners than to eat sugar.

The bottom line: it's fine to use artificial sweeteners, and, in fact, if you are overweight it is healthier to use artificial sweeteners rather than sugar. Today aspartame (NutraSweet) is probably the best choice except for baked goods (since aspartame breaks down at high temperatures). For baked goods use sucralose (Splenda).

Alcohol and Wine

Alcohol abuse is a major source of death, disease, and social and economic loss in the United States. The leading causes of death from alcohol are cirrhosis of the liver, motor vehicle accidents, homicide, and suicide.[234] Alcohol has also been associated with cancers of the mouth, pharynx, larynx, esophagus, and breast.[235] It may be associated with cancers of the pancreas and liver, although this is less clear. Needless to say, alcoholic beverages are high in calories.

It is beyond the scope of this book to discuss all the problems associated with alcohol. One good first step is for individuals with an alcohol problem or family members of such individuals to talk with their doctor.

How much alcohol is too much?[236]
For women: more than 1 drink per day
For men: more than 2 drinks per day

1 drink is defined as a 12 ounce bottle of beer, a 4 ounce glass of wine, 1 ½ ounces of 80 proof spirits, or 1 ounce of 100 proof spirits.

It turns out that drinking *in moderation* may have health benefits. People who have one drink a day have a lower death rate than people who don't drink at all.[237,238,239] (Of course, people who regularly have more than a few drinks a day have a much higher death rate.) Men who have a drink three to seven times a week have a 35% lower risk of heart disease.[240]

Having one drink a day also lowers your risk of dementia.[241,242] Of course, heavy alcohol consumption causes severe dementia.

Red wine contains natural plant molecules called catechins and resveratrol, and these *may* prevent cancer, although this is questionable.[243]

In any event, drinking one glass of red wine three to seven times a week would seem to lengthen your life—although this is still debated in the medical community.

It is important to remember that alcohol consumption by pregnant women causes severe birth defects.[244] Pregnant women or women who may become pregnant should not consume alcohol at all. It is probably a good idea for nursing mothers to avoid alcohol, since alcohol can be passed to the baby in the mother's milk.[245]

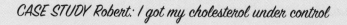

CASE STUDY Robert: I got my cholesterol under control

I am a physician, and I have always been in good health. Heart disease does not run in my family. So I was surprised when I started having chest pains when I walk. I was only 50 and did not expect to have a heart problem.

I went to my physician, and he did some tests. I did a treadmill test, and they did an angiogram, where they take a picture of the arteries in the heart. It turned out I had blockages in the coronary arteries. They did an angioplasty and placed a stent in to keep the arteries open.

I felt better for 6 months but then the chest pains came back. They repeated the angiogram. The stent was developing a blockage.

I had open heart surgery. I tell you, I have never been so scared in my life. But I had one of the best heart surgeons, and everything went great.

I had a long talk with my cardiologist, who's also fantastic. He told me my LDL cholesterol was 190—much higher than normal. I needed to get my cholesterol much lower.

My cardiologist put me on a medication called Lipitor to lower my LDL cholesterol. I take Lipitor every night. My cardiologist also told me I needed to change my diet. That's when I started the Golden Gate Diet.

I am pretty strict in sticking to the Golden Gate Diet. What I really like about the Golden Gate Diet is that it's all healthy food and it's so easy to follow. It gives you another option for everything.

I know the Golden Gate Diet says you can have red meat once in while, but I've cut it out completely. I don't care. I can have fish instead. I have fish at least 3 times a week. Fish has *omega*-3 fatty acids, which protect the heart. I also have chicken, but I cut the skin off.

I cut out all milk products except for skim milk products. I eat nonfat yogurt and skim milk cheese.

I don't eat whole eggs any more. I have egg whites or Eggbeaters. I've found they taste much better if you mix in skim milk cheese and a splash of skim milk.

I don't eat regular peanut butter any more. I eat natural peanut butter which doesn't have partially hydrogenated oils. You just need to mix it up with a knife after you open the jar.

continued..

I eat mashed potatoes. I know the Golden Gate Diet lets you have some made with regular milk, but I have them made with skim milk or water. I eat corn that I get fresh in the grocery store.

I eat pasta. I like penne with marinara sauce. I've found that the penne with ridges is easy to make—it never comes out soggy.

I have a glass of red wine every night at dinner. A drink a day lowers the risk of the heart disease coming back.

I eat with other doctors often. When I go to restaurants I usually have fish. Occasionally I'll have chicken, and I have the waiter tell the chef to cut the skin off. I order a soup and a salad and skip the bread. If the portions are really large, I don't eat everything on my plate. I do try to eat all the vegetables though. If I'm full I skip dessert and just have coffee. If I do have dessert, I eat a slice of pie, or I have them bring me mixed berries.

I am very satisfied with how the food in the Golden Gate Diet tastes.

I have my LDL cholesterol checked regularly. It's been in the 80s, but since I've already had a cardiac bypass, my cardiologist is adjusting my medication to get it under 70.

I didn't go on the Golden Gate Diet to lose weight—I did it to lower my cholesterol. But weight loss has been a side benefit. I'm 5 foot 11 and used to weigh 190 pounds—I now weigh 150.

I feel healthier today than I felt 10 years ago!

Chapter 8

Special Situations:

Children, Pregnancy, Diabetes, Smoking

Weight and Children

Many children in America eat too much. Because they are growing, children do need to consume more calories pound for pound than adults do. That said, obesity is a problem for many children. Every child's pediatrician should calculate and plot the BMI yearly, and children who are overweight or at risk for becoming overweight should change their diet.[246]

In adults a BMI greater than 30 indicates being obese. In children, it's a little different. The BMIs corresponding to being overweight and to being at risk for becoming overweight in children change with age. Pediatricians use tables called BMI-for-age to determine if a child is overweight or at risk for becoming overweight.[247,248,249]

Children and adolescents are at risk for becoming overweight if their BMI-for-age is greater than the 85th percentile on the tables. Children and adolescents are overweight if their BMI-for-age is greater than the 95th percentile on the tables.

For example, a 5 year old girl with a BMI of 22 would be above the curve, so she would be considered overweight.

Young children have much less muscle than adults do, so it is not surprising that the 95th percentile for a 5 year old girl would be a BMI of 18, while 95th percentile for a 20 year old woman would be a BMI of 32.

The tables were developed from national surveys conducted by the CDC between 1963 and 1994. Since then children in America have gotten much heavier. However, pediatricians consider a child today overweight if the child is greater than 95th percentile on the following tables.

So between 1963 and 1994 5% of children were overweight. But, sadly, the percentage of children who are overweight has tripled since then to about 15%.[250]

The recommendations in this book as to what foods are healthy to eat will work for children as well as for adults. Children should be actively involved in choosing a healthy diet rather than having their diet dictated to them by their parents! Offer children choices of healthy foods, then let them choose which healthy foods they want to eat.

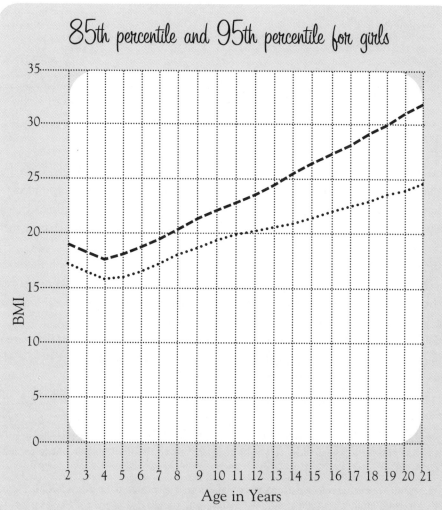

85th percentile and 95th percentile of BMI-for-age in girls. Data from the National Center for Health Statistics, CDC (Centers for Disease Control and Prevention). For a more detailed BMI-for-age chart for girls go to: www.cdc.gov/nchs/data/nhanes/growthcharts/set1clinical/cj41c024.pdf

•••••••• 85th percentile

▬ ▬ ▬ ▬ 95th percentile

For children who do need to lose weight, it is important that their diets be coordinated with their pediatricians.

Children should participate in physical activity and active play. Television watching should be limited to a maximum of 2 hours a day.

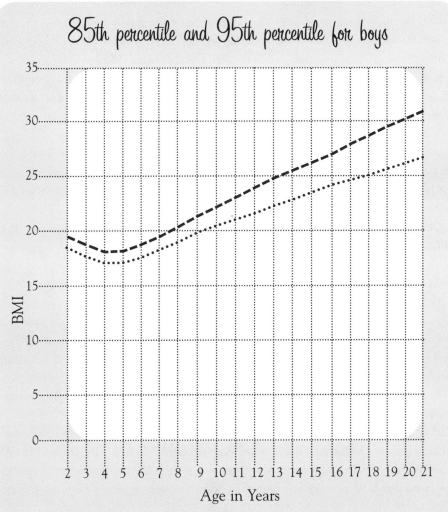

85th percentile and 95th percentile for boys

Age in Years

85th percentile and 95th percentile of BMI-for-age in girls. Data from the National Center for Health Statistics, CDC (Centers for Disease Control and Prevention). For a more detailed BMI-for-age chart for girls go to:
www.cdc.gov/nchs/data/nhanes/growthcharts/set1clinical/cj41c024.pdf

.... 85th percentile

- - - - - 95th percentile

Weight Loss, Health, Pregnancy, and Nursing

Pregnant women, of course, need to eat more since they are eating for two. Obesity, however, is a major health problem in pregnant women.

Women who are overweight or obese have a greater risk of disease during pregnancy, both for themselves and their fetus, than normal weight women have.[251] Babies of obese women are at increased risk of dying during infancy. Even women who are moderately overweight are at increased risk for diabetes and blood pressure disorders during pregnancy, and obese women are at even higher risk. Blood pressure disorders during pregnancy can be very serious and occasionally result in the death of either the mother or her baby. Overweight women have a higher rate of Cesarean delivery and are at increased risk for complications after delivery. Babies of obese women are at increased risk for abnormally large size at delivery, which can result in "shoulder dystocia"—nerve damage to the baby's arm nerves. Babies of obese women are also at risk for spinal cord defects.

Overweight or obese pregnant women need to coordinate any weight loss plan with their obstetricians, since it is important to maintain adequate nutrition for the fetus.

There are several specific things in terms of diet that a pregnant woman can do to maintain her baby's health.

Avoid alcohol

Alcohol consumption by pregnant women can result in their children having the fetal alcohol syndrome. Children with the fetal alcohol syndrome have decreased IQ,[252] a number of deformities including facial deformities, retarded growth,[253,254] and behavioral disorders.[255]

Fetal alcohol syndrome is only the most dramatic presentation of alcohol consumption by pregnant women.

Does moderate drinking during pregnancy lower a child's IQ? To examine this question, researchers conducted a study of 482 children aged 7 ? years. This controlled study found that the children of women who drank as few as 2 drinks a day during pregnancy had an average IQ 7 points lower than the children of women who did not drink during pregnancy.[256]

I advise women who are pregnant or who are likely to become pregnant to avoid alcohol completely.

CASE STUDY Jenny: I gained weight during pregnancy and couldn't lose it—
until I tried the Golden Gate Diet

When I was pregnant with my daughter Sarah, I gained 30 pounds. One year later, I had not lost the weight. I'm 5'7", and at 170 pounds I did not look or feel right. I spent a lot of money going to a weight loss program, but it didn't seem to help.

Then Dr. Brook put me on the Golden Gate Diet. I was really happy to find a doctor who knew about weight loss and was more interested in me than in my pocketbook!

I liked the fact that the diet is scientifically based and that Dr. Brook has undergone training both as a doctor and as a scientist. I also liked the fact that the diet makes good sense. You eat bulky food, and that stretches your stomach and tells your brain you're not hungry any more. It makes a lot more sense to me than this low-carb stuff.

I started on the 1200 calories a day meal plan. Every time I started feeling hungry it was already time to eat again—either a meal or a snack between meals. It was very easy to do. I liked the fact that I was eating healthy foods.

I am an excellent cook, and the meal plan let me cook food that tastes good. For dinner, we might have veal cutlet or baked tuna or roasted skinless chicken breast. The meals really do not take very long to prepare.

After 4 months, I lost 30 pounds. The best part is, I've kept the weight off.

My husband was very supportive of me in my dieting. He ate the same foods I did. He was not trying to lose weight, but he lost 15 pounds. I like the fact that I know that with the Golden Gate Diet we are eating healthy food.

Take a folic acid supplement

There is good evidence that folic acid decreases the risks of spina bifida and certain other disorders of spinal cord development. Spina bifida is a disorder in which the spinal cord fails to close and is the most common permanently disabling birth defect. Spina bifida and these other disorders are called neural tube defects. The neural tube is the developmental precursor of the brain and spinal cord in the embryo, and all these disorders occur as a result of failure of the neural tube to close.

The risk of neural tube disorders occurring is greatly reduced by taking a folic acid supplement. A conclusive study of at-risk women found that taking a pill of 4 mg of folic acid a day reduced the risk of having a child with a neural tube defect by 72%.[257] Since half of all pregnancies in this country are unplanned, it is recommended that all women of child-bearing age take 400 micrograms of folic acid a day.[258] Most multi-vitamin pills contain 400 micrograms of folic acid.

How much folic acid should women who are pregnant or are trying to become pregnant take? The higher the folic acid dose is, the lower the risk of spina bifida and other neural tube disorders. It has been estimated that the infants of women who take 400 micrograms of folic acid a day have a 36% lower risk of spina bifida than the infants of women who do not take any folic acid supplement, that the infants of women who take 1 mg of folic acid a day have a 57% lower risk of spina bifida, and that the infants of women who take 5 mg of folic acid a day have an 85% lower risk of spina bifida.[259] However, some physicians are concerned that taking folic acid may mask or even exacerbate vitamin B_{12} deficiency.[260] My advice: pregnant women and women who are trying to become pregnant who are not at-risk should take a folic acid supplement of 1000 micrograms a day (400 micrograms in a multi-vitamin pill plus an additional 600 micrograms).

Natural sources of folic acid include vegetables (especially dark green, leafy vegetables), fruits, beans, whole grains, and breakfast cereals. It is possible to consume 1000 micrograms a day of folic acid from food. However, there is no downside for pregnant women to take 1000 micrograms of folic acid from a combination of a multi-vitamin and a folic acid supplement, and I think it is wise, since this way a pregnant can be certain she is consuming that much folic acid.

At-risk women should take 5 mg of folic acid a day under the supervision of their doctors.

Breastfeeding.

Breastfeeding is a subject that people having strong feelings about. Human milk contains antibodies and white blood cells, which prevent infection in the infant. These factors are not present in cow's milk or formula. Compared with bottle-fed infants, breastfed infants have lower rates of certain infectious diseases, and when they do contract these infections, the course is often less severe than the course in bottle-fed infants.

The American Academy of Pediatrics Section on Breastfeeding has recommended that infants be exclusively breastfed until 6 months of age (i.e. that infants in the first 6 months of life be fed only breast milk unless there is a specific reason why the mother cannot or should not breastfeed).[261] In addition, they have recommended that infants continue to be breastfed from 6 months to 1 year, but that during this time the infants should be introduced to other foods, particularly iron-rich foods. They also have recommended that breastfeeding infants receive a daily supplement of 200 IU of vitamin D until such time as the infants are taking 500 ml of vitamin D-fortified milk or formula.

It is difficult for many women who lead busy lives and who work to breastfeed for the length of time advocated by the American Academy of Pediatrics. The decision of whether or not to breastfeed is a highly personal one that every woman needs to make for herself.

Surprisingly, there is nothing else that has been conclusively proven in terms of maternal diet to improve a baby's health. (Although obviously you should avoid toxic substances and should discuss all medications with your doctor as certain medications can cause birth defects.) The bottom line seems to be that sufficient but not excessive nutrition is what is needed for a healthy baby, rather than specific foods.

Diabetes

Diabetes is a disorder of sugar metabolism. There are two types of diabetes, type 1 and type 2. In type 1 diabetes, the immune system destroys the insulin-producing cells in the pancreas. In type 2 diabetes, cells throughout the body resist the action of insulin.

The vast majority of adults with diabetes have type 2 diabetes. In children, type 1 diabetes is more common than type 2 diabetes.

The more overweight you are, the greater your risk of getting type 2 diabetes. At the extreme, very obese (BMI 40) people are 20 times more likely to get diabetes than normal weight people (BMI less than 25).[221] Modest weight loss reduces the incidence of diabetes by 40–60%;[222] in the remaining patients who are not completely cured, modest weight loss reduces the severity of their diabetes.

Though losing weight is by far the best way to avoid type 2 diabetes and to cure or to reduce the severity of diabetes if you have diabetes, eating cereal fiber and whole grain foods is helpful as well. As was discussed above in chapter 7, for people of a given weight, people who eat a large amount of cereal fiber have a 30% lower risk of developing type 2 diabetes than people who eat little cereal fiber, and people who eat a large amount of whole grain foods have a 30–40% lower risk of diabetes than people who eat a small amount of whole grain foods.

It used to be thought that sugar was particularly unhealthy for people with diabetes. Specifically, it was believed that when people with diabetes ate sugar, their blood sugar level would increase to very high levels. Many studies of diabetes have been done, and it has been proven that people with diabetes can eat sugar-containing foods safely. A panel of physicians with expertise in diabetes assembled by the American Diabetes Association concluded that eating sugar in normal amounts does not impair blood glucose control in people with type 1 or type 2 diabetes. [264] Thus, people with diabetes can eat sugar-containing foods. Of course, many (but not all) sugar-containing foods have a high caloric density, and these should be avoided by people with diabetes who are trying to lose weight!

The bottom line: you can reduce your risk of type 2 diabetes dramatically by losing weight. If you have type 2 diabetes, it can be made less severe and often cured by losing weight. Eating cereal fiber and whole grain foods is also helpful in reducing the risk of type 2 diabetes.

CASE STUDY Armando: my diabetes melted away

I'm 55, and I was overweight. I am 5'6" tall, and I weighed 200 pounds. I have had diabetes for the last 10 years, and I took Glucophage to control my diabetes.

My doctor told me I needed to lose weight. I had been trying to lose weight for the last 10 years. I would lose a few pounds, but I would gain them back soon. My doctor had told me to avoid foods with sugars. That meant no sweets and also no fruit.

A few years ago I started developing pain in my left leg during walking. I run a contracting business, and I need to get around in my job. The pain was interfering with my work.

Dr. Brook is a tough guy, but he's a good doctor. He told me I was developing blockages in the leg arteries. He said that if I didn't change my diet and lose weight, I might need an operation to bypass the blockages in my leg arteries. I appreciate his being honest with me.

I told him, "Doctor, you don't understand, in my family we like to eat." He put me on the Golden Gate Diet.

It took a little getting used to, but I understand now what foods I can eat and what foods I can't eat.

Some things surprised me a bit. Dr. Brook said that I could eat fruit. In fact, he said I should eat lots of fruits and vegetables. It wouldn't make my diabetes worse. The only thing that mattered was losing weight.

I eat cereal or oatmeal for breakfast every morning. I like Raisin Bran cereal. I don't eat any cereal with *trans*-fats.

For lunch I usually take a sandwich to work with me. I usually have a salad as well.

Dinner is my favorite. We have a lot of chicken (without the skin) and a

continued..

lot of fish. I am used to eating spicy foods, and the Golden Gate Diet lets me eat spicy foods. I even have dessert most of the time. I have a healthy dessert like chocolate pudding or fruit. Sometimes I have apple pie.

I guess a lot of the food I had been eating was processed food, not the natural foods I should have been eating. I also understand that not all natural foods are healthy. I gave up red meat and all the snack foods. I also had been eating some fast foods—I don't go to McDonald's anymore.

Dr. Brook put me on an exercise program. I would walk until I would develop leg pain. Every day I could walk a little farther before I started getting pain. Dr. Brook also sent me to an excellent podiatrist. I am very careful about how I treat my feet now.

The Golden Gate Diet really made a difference. Within months I lost 40 pounds. My diabetes melted away! I don't need to take the Glucophage any more. I still get leg pains sometimes when I walk a long distance, but it's much better.

I know I've got to take care of myself. I can't quit. I have to eat healthy for the rest of my life. I don't have a choice. I am not going to lose my leg.

Dr. Brook really helped me.

Smoking and Weight Loss

Many people who smoke are afraid to quit in part because they are afraid they will gain weight when they quit. While it is true you may gain some weight after quitting smoking, smoking is such a dangerous addiction that it is better to quit smoking and gain some pounds than to continue smoking. Smoking is a leading cause of heart disease, cancer, and stroke.[265,266] It has been estimated that half of all smokers die from tobacco use.

There are many methods to quit smoking, such as smoking-cessation programs, nicotine-replacement pills, and the nicotine patch. It is beyond the scope of this book to discuss how to quit smoking, but one way to start is to discuss quitting with your doctor.

The best way to proceed is to quit smoking first before you start dieting.[267] After you have quit smoking, then try to lose weight. But don't continue smoking and not diet—your risk of heart disease if you smoke and are overweight or obese is extremely high.

Chapter 9

What Foods to Eat,
and what Foods not to Eat

This chapter includes charts telling you exactly what foods to eat and what foods not to eat. I created these charts using raw data on the composition of foods from the Agricultural Research Service of the United States Department of Agriculture.[268] Of course, the recommendation whether or not to eat a particular food comes from me, not from the USDA!

All other things being equal, I have listed solid food with a caloric density less than 2 and liquids with a caloric density less than 0.4 as helping weight loss. The lower the caloric density, in general, the more a food will promote weight loss—thus eating solid foods with a caloric density less than 1 will cause faster weight loss than solid foods with a caloric density of 2. Liquids have a stricter standard since an equivalent weight of liquids will be less likely to make you feel full than the same weight of solid foods. This is because liquids can pass through the stomach and intestines more quickly than solid foods.

Most of the foods that Americans eat are included in the tables that follow. The easiest thing to do to figure out the caloric density of a food is to just look in the tables that follow. If you would like to calculate the caloric density on your own, it's not hard though: just divide the calories by the weight in grams.

Caloric density = calories ÷ weight (in grams)

For example, the average peach has 40 calories and weighs 100 grams. It's easy to calculate the caloric density:

Caloric density = 40 calories ÷ 100 grams = 0.4

While the caloric density determines whether a food will cause you to gain weight or to lose weight, there are other things to consider in deciding whether a food is healthy or unhealthy. For example, whole eggs have a caloric density of 1.5, and eating whole eggs will help you lose weight. However, whole eggs are loaded with saturated fat and cholesterol and will increase the risk of heart disease: so whole eggs are not a healthy food and not part of the Golden Gate Diet.

So the decision about whether a food is healthy or unhealthy depends not only on its caloric density but on other factors as well, such as the amount of saturated fat the food contains.

The healthy foods of the Golden Gate Diet are shaded black. Unhealthy foods are shaded blue. There are a few foods, like nuts, that will cause you to gain weight but are part of the Golden Gate Diet since they cut your risk of heart disease dramatically. (Just don't overdo it while you're trying to lose pounds!)

Beverages

Alcohol

Feel free to enjoy a glass of red wine. A glass of red wine 3 to 7 times a week may even lengthen your life. White table wine and light beer are also good to drink in moderation. (But don't have one glass of red wine, one glass of white wine, *and* one light beer every day!) Stay away from regular beer, hard liquor, and dessert wine: these all are high in calories.

Carbonated Beverages

Stick to diet soda sweetened with aspartame and club soda. A glass of ginger ale once in a while is alright. Stay away from non-diet soda: it is high in calories.

Beverage	Suggested Consumption	Caloric density (Cal/g)	Amount	Calories
club soda	yes	0.0	12 fl oz	0
cola	no	0.4	12 fl oz	152
diet cola	yes	0.0	12 fl oz	4
ginger ale	in moderation	0.3	12 fl oz	124
grape soda	no	0.4	12 fl oz	160
lemon lime soda	no	0.4	12 fl oz	147
orange soda	no	0.5	12 fl oz	179
pepper soda	no	0.4	12 fl oz	151
root beer	no	0.4	12 fl oz	152

Coffee and Cocoa

It is fine to drink coffee—it has very few calories in it. But don't put a lot of sugar or cream in it!

Cocoa is high in calories and best avoided. Cocoa sweetened with aspartame and that contains nonfat dry milk (and that is prepared with water or skim milk but *not* fat-containing milk) is alright.

Beverage	Amount	Suggested Consumption	Caloric density (Cal/g)	Calories
brewed coffee	6 fl oz	yes	0.0	4
espresso	2 fl oz	yes	0.1	5
instant coffee	6 fl oz	yes	0.0	4
cocoa powder*	1 oz	no	0.5	03
cocoa powder**	1 serving	in moderation	0.3	48

* containing nonfat dry milk, prepared with 6 oz water
** 1 envelope mix containing nonfat dry milk and aspartame prepared with 6 oz water

Fruit Drinks

Stay away from fruit drinks—they are high in calories. If you want to drink lemonade, drink lemonade that is sweetened with aspartame.

Tea

Tea has almost no calories and a caloric density close to 0. Of course, don't add a lot of cream and sugar. Choose tea sweetened with NutraSweet instead.

Water

It's a good idea to drink water—it has no calories and thus a caloric density of 0. Drinking water instead of soda or juice will reduce the number of calories you are taking in.

Dairy Products

Cheese

Cheeses—even so-called "low fat" cheeses made with part-skim milk—are high in saturated fat and best avoided. The exceptions are nonfat cheeses, which are good to eat. If you have salt-sensitive high blood pressure, be aware that cheeses are high in sodium.

Dressing	Amount	Suggested Consumption	Caloric density (Cal/g)	Calories
cheese natural blue	1 oz	no	3.6	100
cheese Camembert	1 wedge	no	3.0	114
cheddar cheese cut pieces	1 oz	no	4.1	114
cheddar cheese cut pieces	1 cubic "	no	4.0	68
cheddar cheese shredded	1 cup	no	4.0	455
cottage cheese 4% fat large curd	1 cup	no	1.0	233
cottage cheese 4% fat small curd	1 cup	no	1.0	217
cottage cheese 4% fat with fruit	1 cup	no	1.2	279
cottage cheese 2% fat	1 cup	no	0.9	203
cottage cheese 1% fat	1 cup	yes	0.7	164
cottage cheese less than ½% fat (uncreamed)	1 cup	yes	0.9	123
cream cheese regular	1 oz	no	3.5	99
cream cheese regular	1 tbsp	no	3.4	51
cream cheese low fat	1 tbsp	no	2.3	35
cream cheese fat free	1 tbsp	yes	0.9	15
feta cheese	1 tbsp	no	4.7	75
cheddar or colby cheese low fat	1 oz	no	1.8	49
mozzarella cheese whole milk	1 oz	no	2.9	80
mozarella cheese part skim milk	1 oz	no	2.8	79
muenster cheese	1 oz	no	3.7	104
neufchatel cheese	1 oz	no	2.6	74
parmesan cheese grated	1 cup	no	4.6	456
parmesan cheese grated	1 tbsp	no	4.6	23
parmesan cheese grated	1 oz	no	4.6	129
provolone cheese	1 oz	no	3.6	100
ricotta cheese whole milk	1 cup	no	1.7	428
ricotta cheese part skim milk	1 cup	no	1.4	340
Swiss cheese	1 oz	no	3.8	107
American cheese regular	1 oz	no	3.8	106
American cheese fat free	1 slice	yes	1.5	31
Swiss cheese processed	1 oz	no	3.4	95
American cheese food	1 oz	no	3.3	93
American cheese spread	1 oz	no	2.9	82

Cream

Cream is high in saturated fat and should be avoided. Nonfat sour cream and imitation liquid creamer are a better idea.

Ice Cream, Sherbet, and Frozen Yogurt

When ice cream, sherbet, sorbet, and frozen yogurt reach the stomach, they melt, and pass rapidly out of the stomach. So they don't make you feel full for long, and they have a lot of calories. The caloric densities of ice cream, sherbet, sorbet, and frozen yogurt are very high for liquids—and since they melt rapidly, they should be compared with liquids. For example, the caloric density of chocolate ice cream is 2.2. That's more than 5 times higher than the cut-off for liquids of 0.4. What's more, full-fat ice cream, sherbet, and frozen yogurt are high in saturated fat: avoid them. If you want to lose weight, even sorbet and nonfat ice cream, sherbet, and frozen yogurt should be only for a special occasion.

Milk

Avoid whole milk—it is high in saturated fat. Drink skim milk instead—it is a good source of protein and calcium. Drink 1% fat milk and buttermilk only in moderation.

Yogurt

Yogurt is a healthy food that is high in protein and calcium. Eat especially nonfat yogurt. You can also eat low fat yogurt with added fruit. Stay away from yogurt made from whole milk—it is high in saturated fat.

Yogurt	Amount	Suggested Consumption	Caloric density (Cal/g)	Calories
lowfat yogurt with added fruit	1 cup	yes	1.0	231
plain lowfat yogurt	1 cup	no	0.6	144
nonfat yogurt with added fruit	1 cup	yes	0.9	213
plain nonfat yogurt	1 cup	yes	0.6	127
whole milk yogurt	1 cup	no	0.6	139
nonfat yogurt with low calorie sweetener	1 cup	yes	0.4	98

Eggs

Egg whites are a great source of protein and can be prepared in many different ways. You can also eat egg substitutes (for example, Eggbeaters). Stay away from whole eggs—egg yolk is high in saturated fat and cholesterol.

Butter and margarine

Butter and margarine are extremely high in calories and should not be eaten. Butter is very high in saturated fat, and margarine is very high in *trans*-fat. For cooking, use vegetable oil instead.

Oils

Oils are extremely high in calories and caloric density. Use them in moderation. Stay away from hydrogenated and partially hydrogenated oils.

Salad dressings

Regular salad dressing and mayonnaise are high in calories and should not be eaten. Instead you may eat any low calorie salad dressing (except low calorie blue cheese dressing which is high in saturated fat). Use nonfat mayonnaise instead of light mayonnaise, which is relatively high in calories and saturated fat.

Dressing	Amount	Suggested Consumption	Caloric density (Cal/g)	Calories
blue cheese*	1 tbsp	no	5.1	77
blue cheese**	1 tbsp	no	1.0	15
Caesar*	1 tbsp	no	5.2	78
Caesar**	1 tbsp	in moderation	1.1	17
French*	1 tbsp	no	4.2	67
French**	1 tbsp	in moderation	1.4	22
Italian*	1 tbsp	no	4.6	69
Italian**	1 tbsp	in moderation	1.1	16
mayonnaise*	1 tbsp	no	7.1	99
mayonnaise**	1 tbsp	no	3.3	49
mayonnaise***	1 tbsp	in moderation	0.8	12
Russian*	1 tbsp	no	5.1	76
Russian**	1 tbsp	in moderation	1.4	23
Thousand*	1 tbsp	no	3.7	59
Thousand island**	1 tbsp	in moderation	1.6	24
vinegar and oil	1 tbsp	no	4.4	70
vinegar	1 tbsp	yes	0.1	2

* regular   ** low calorie   *** nonfat

Fish and Shellfish

Fish and shellfish are healthy, low in calories, and high in protein. Baked and broiled fish have fewer calories than breaded, fried fish. Avoid swordfish—it is high in mercury.

What Foods to Eat, and What Foods Not to Eat

Seafood	Amount	Suggested Consumption	Caloric density (Cal/g)	Calories
catfish, breaded, fried	6 oz	no	2.3	390
clam, raw	1 medium	yes	0.7	11
clams, breaded, fried	¾ cup	no	3.9	451
cod, baked or broiled	6 oz	yes	1.0	178
Alaska king crab steamed	6 oz	in moderation	1.0	164
imitation crab	6 oz	in moderation	1.0	174
blue crab, steamed	6 oz	yes	1.0	174
canned crabmeat	1 cup	yes	1.0	134
crab cake with egg, fried	1 cake	yes	1.6	93
fish fillet battered, fried	1 fillet	in moderation	2.3	211
fish stick, breaded	1 stick	in moderation	2.7	76
flounder or sole, baked or broiled	6 oz	yes	1.2	198
haddock, baked or broiled	6 oz	yes	1.1	190
halibut, baked or broiled	6 oz	yes	1.4	238
herring, pickled	6 oz	in moderation	2.6	446
lobster, steamed	6 oz	yes	1.0	166
ocean perch, baked or broiled	6 oz	yes	1.2	206
oysters, raw	6 medium	yes	0.7	57
oysters, breaded, fried	6 oz	no	2.0	334
pollock, baked or broiled	6 oz	yes	1.1	192
rockfish, baked or broiled	6 oz	yes	1.2	206
orange roughy, baked or broiled	6 oz	yes	0.9	152
salmon, baked or broiled	6 oz	yes	2.2	368
canned pink salmon, (with bones)	6 oz	yes	1.4	236
smoked salmon	6 oz	in moderation	1.2	198
canned sardines in oil (with bones)	6 oz	yes	2.1	354
scallops, breaded, fried	6 large	yes	2.2	200
scallops, steamed	6 oz	yes	1.1	190
shrimp, breaded, fried	6 oz	in moderation	2.4	412
shrimp, canned	6 oz	yes	1.2	204
swordfish, baked or broiled	6 oz	limit	1.6	264
trout, baked or broiled	6 oz	yes	1.7	288
tuna, baked or broiled	6 oz	yes	1.4	236
tuna, chunk light, in oil	6 oz	yes	2.0	336
tuna, chunk light, in water	6 oz	yes	1.2	198
tuna, solid white albacore, in water	6 oz	yes	1.3	218
tuna salad: light tuna in oil, mayonnaise	1 cup	yes	1.9	383

Fruit and Fruit Juices

Eating fruit is good for you—fruit are low in calories and will help you lose weight. Try to have 4 servings of fruit every day. How big is a serving? About the size of a medium-sized apple, banana, orange, or pear, or a ½ cup of chopped, cooked, or canned fruit. Go easy on the fruit juices—they have a fair amount of calories and won't fill you up the way solid fruit will. Fruit is also a good source of fiber.

Fruit and Fruit Juices	Amount	Suggested Consumption	Caloric density (Cal/g)	Calories
apples	1 apple	yes	0.6	81
dried apples	5 rings	in moderation	2.4	78
apple juice	1 cup	in moderation	0.5	117
apple pie filling	⅛ of 21-oz can	yes	1.0	75
sweetened applesauce	1 cup	yes	0.8	194
unsweetened applesauce	1 cup	yes	0.4	105
apricots	1 apricot	yes	0.5	17
apricots in syrup	1 cup	yes	0.8	214
apricots in juice	1 cup	yes	0.5	117
dried apricots	10 halves	yes	2.4	83
apricot nectar	1 cup	in moderation	0.6	141
Asian pear	1 pear	yes	0.4	116
California avocado	1 oz	in moderation	1.8	50
Florida avocado	1 oz	in moderation	1.1	32
whole bananas	1 banana	yes	0.9	109
sliced bananas	1 cup	yes	0.9	138
blackberries	1 cup	yes	0.5	75
raw blueberries	1 cup	yes	0.6	81
frozen blueberries	1 cup	yes	0.8	186
carambola (starfruit)	1 fruit	yes	0.3	30
sour cherries canned	1 cup	yes	0.4	88
sweet cherries	10 cherries	yes	0.7	49
cherry pie filling	⅕ of 21 oz can	yes	1.2	85
dried sweetened cranberries	¼ cup	no	3.3	92
sweetened cranberry sauce	1 slice	yes	1.5	86
whole dates	5 dates	yes	2.8	116
dried figs	2 figs	yes	2.6	97

continued..

Fruit and Fruit Juices	Amount	Suggested Consumption	Caloric density (Cal/g)	Calories
fruit cocktail in syrup	1 cup	yes	0.7	181
fruit cocktail in juice	1 cup	yes	0.5	109
pink grapefruit	½ grapefruit	yes	0.3	37
white grapefruit	½ grapefruit	yes	0.3	39
canned grapefruit in light syrup	1 cup	yes	0.6	152
pink grapefruit juice	1 cup	in moderation	0.4	96
white grapefruit juice	1 cup	in moderation	0.4	96
unsweetened canned grapefruit juice	1 cup	in moderation	0.4	94
sweetened canned grapefruit juice	1 cup	in moderation	0.5	115
grapefruit juice from concentrate	1 cup	in moderation	0.4	101
seedless grapes	10 grapes	yes	0.7	36
grape juice	1 cup	in moderation	0.6	154
grape juice from concentrated	1 cup	in moderation	0.5	128
kiwi	1 medium	yes	0.6	46
lemons	1 lemon	yes	0.3	17
lemon juice raw	juice of 1 lemon	yes	0.3	12
canned lemon juice unsweetened	1 tbsp	yes	0.2	3
raw lime juice	juice of 1 lime	yes	0.3	10
canned lime juice unsweetened	1 tbsp	yes	0.2	3
mangos	1 mango	yes	0.7	135
cantaloupe	⅛ melon	yes	0.4	24
honeydew	⅛ melon	yes	0.4	56
mixed fruit frozen sweetened	1 cup	yes	1.0	245
nectarines	1 nectarine	yes	0.5	67
oranges	1 orange	yes	0.5	62
orange juice, raw	1 cup	in moderation	0.5	112
orange juice, canned, unsweetened	1 cup	in moderation	0.4	105
orange juice, chilled (refrigerator case)	1 cup	in moderation	0.4	110

continued..

Fruit and Fruit Juices	Amount	Suggested Consumption	Caloric density (Cal/g)	Calories
orange juice from concentrate	1 cup	in moderation	0.5	112
papaya	1 papaya	yes	0.4	119
peaches	1 peach	yes	0.4	42
peaches in heavy syrup	1 cup	yes	0.7	194
peaches in juice	1 cup	yes	0.4	109
dried peaches	3 halves	yes	2.4	93
frozen peaches	1 cup	yes	0.9	235
pears	1 pear	yes	0.6	98
pears in heavy syrup	1 cup	yes	0.7	197
pears in juice	1 cup	yes	0.5	124
pineapple	1 cup	yes	0.5	76
pineapple in heavy syrup	1 cup	yes	0.8	198
pineapple in juice	1 cup	yes	0.6	149
pineapple juice unsweetened	1 cup	no	0.6	140
plantain cooked	1 cup	yes	1.2	179
plums raw	1 plum	yes	0.6	36
plums in heavy syrup	1 cup	yes	0.9	230
plums in juice	1 cup	yes	0.6	146
prunes uncooked	5 prunes	yes	2.4	100
prunes stewed	1 cup	yes	1.1	265
prune juice	1 cup	no	0.7	182
raisins	1 packet	in moderation	3.0	42
raspberries raw	1 cup	yes	0.5	60
raspberries frozen sweetened	1 cup	yes	1.0	258
rhubarb cooked with sugar	1 cup	yes	1.2	278
strawberries	1 strawberry	yes	0.3	4
strawberries frozen sweetened	1 cup	yes	1.0	245
tangerines raw	1 tangerine	yes	0.4	37
tangerines canned	1 cup	yes	0.6	154
tangerine juice	1 cup	no	0.5	125
watermelon wedge	1 wedge	yes	0.3	92

Grain Products

Bread

Don't eat a lot of bread, since bread is relatively high in calories and caloric density.*
Reduced calorie bread is a good alternative.

Bread	Amount	Suggested Consumption	Caloric density (Cal/g)	Calories
plain bread crumbs	1 cup	no	4.0	427
seasoned bread crumbs	1 cup	no	4.0	440
bread stuffing	½ cup	in moderation	1.8	178
cracked wheat bread	1 slice	in moderation	2.6	65
challah	½" slice	limit	2.9	115
French bread (includes sourdough)	½" slice	limit	2.8	69
Indian fry (Navajo) bread	5" bread	no	3.3	296
Italian bread	1 slice	in moderation	2.7	54
matzoh	1 matzoh	no	4.0	112
mixed grain bread untoasted	1 slice	in moderation	2.5	65
mixed grain bread toasted	1 slice	in moderation	2.7	65
oatmeal bread untoasted	1 slice	in moderation	2.7	73
oatmeal bread toasted	1 slice	limit	2.9	73
pita	6 ½" pita	limit	2.8	165
pumpernickel untoasted	1 slice	in moderation	2.5	80
pumpernickel toasted	1 slice	limit	2.8	80
raisin bread untoasted	1 slice	in moderation	2.7	71
raisin bread toasted	1 slice	limit	3.0	71
dinner rolls	1 roll	no	3.0	84
hamburger or hotdog rolls	1 roll	limit	2.9	123

continued...

* In fairness, bread may be a bit less fattening than its caloric density would lead us to believe, since as bread absorbs liquid in the stomach its non-air volume goes up, and its caloric density goes down. It's OK to have some bread, just don't go crazy.

Bread	Amount	Suggested Consumption	Caloric density (Cal/g)	Calories
hard Kaiser rolls	1 roll	limit	2.9	167
rye bread untoasted	1 slice	in moderation	2.6	83
rye bread toasted	1 slice	limit	2.8	68
rye bread reduced calorie	1 slice	yes	2.0	47
taco shell baked	1 medium	no	4.8	62
corn tortillas ready to cook (6" dia)	1 tortilla	in moderation	2.2	58
flour tortillas ready to cook (6" dia)	1 tortilla	no	3.3	104
wheat bread untoasted	1 slice	in moderation	2.6	65
wheat bread toasted	1 slice	limit	2.8	65
wheat bread reduced calorie	1 slice	yes	2.0	46
white bread untoasted	1 slice	in moderation	2.7	67
white bread toasted	1 slice	limit	2.9	64
white bread reduced calorie	1 slice	yes	2.1	48
whole wheat bread untoasted	1 slice	in moderation	2.5	69
whole wheat bread toasted	1 slice	limit	2.8	69

Cereal

Cereal can be a healthy food and a good source of fiber. Unfortunately, most manufacturers add large amounts of sugar and *trans*-fats to their cereals. What's worse, they advertise their cereals as health foods when in fact they are very fattening and unhealthy. I recommend a few cereals even though they have a high caloric density because they are high in fiber. Stick to cereals that have a low caloric density, that have no *trans*-fats, and that are high in fiber.

Cereal	Amount	Suggested Consumption	Caloric density (Cal/g)	Calories
white corn grits	1 cup	yes	0.6	145
yellow corn grits	1 cup	yes	0.6	145
instant grits	1 packet	yes	0.7	89
regular CREAM OF WHEAT	1 cup	yes	0.5	133
quick CREAM OF WHEAT	1 cup	yes	0.5	129
Mix 'n Eat CREAM OF WHEAT	1 packet	yes	0.7	102
MALT O MEAL	1 cup	yes	0.5	122
regular oatmeal	1 cup	yes	0.6	145
instant oatmeal	1 packet	yes	0.6	104
QUAKER instant oatmeal apples and cinnamon	1 packet	yes	0.8	125
QUAKER instant oatmeal maple and brown sugar	1 packet	yes	1.0	153
WHEATENA	1 cup	yes	0.6	136
ALL BRAN	½ cup	yes	2.6	79
APPLE CINNAMON CHEERIOS	¾ cup	no	3.9	118
APPLE JACKS	1 cup	no	3.9	116
BASIC 4	1 cup	no	3.7	201
BERRY BERRY KIX	¾ cup	no	4.0	120
CAP'N CRUNCH	¾ cup	no	4.0	107
CAP'N CRUNCH'S CRUNCHBERRIES	¾ cup	no	4.0	104
CAP'N CRUNCH'S PEANUT BUTTER CRUNCH	¾ cup	no	4.2	112
CHEERIOS	1 cup	no	3.7	110
CORN CHEX	1 cup	no	3.8	113
HONEY NUT CHEX	¾ cup	no	3.9	117
MULTI BRAN CHEX	1 cup	yes	3.4	165
RICE CHEX	1 ¼ cup	no	3.8	117
WHEAT CHEX	1 cup	no	3.5	104
CINNAMON LIFE	1 cup	no	3.8	190
CINNAMON TOAST CRUNCH	¾ cup	no	4.1	124
COCOA KRISPIES	¾ cup	no	3.9	120
COCOA PUFFS	1 cup	no	4.0	119
GENERAL MILLS CORN FLAKES	1 ⅓ cup	no	3.7	112
KELLOGG'S CORN FLAKES	1 cup	no	3.6	102

continued..

Cereal	Amount	Suggested Consumption	Caloric density (Cal/g)	Calories
CORN POPS	1 cup	no	3.8	118
CRISPIX	1 cup	no	3.7	108
FROOT LOOPS	1 cup	no	3.9	117
FROSTED FLAKES	¾ cup	no	3.8	119
FROSTED MINI WHEATS REGULAR	1 cup	no	3.4	173
FROSTED MINI WHEATS BITE SIZE	1 cup	no	3.4	187
GOLDEN GRAHAMS	¾ cup	no	3.9	116
HONEY FROSTED WHEATIES	¾ cup	no	3.7	110
HONEY NUT CHEERIOS	1 cup	no	3.8	115
HONEY NUT CLUSTERS	1 cup	no	3.9	213
KIX	1⅓ cup	no	3.8	114
LIFE	¾ cup	no	3.8	121
LUCKY CHARMS	1 cup	no	3.9	116
NATURE VALLEY GRANOLA	¾ cup	no	4.5	248
PRODUCT 19	1 cup	no	3.7	110
puffed rice	1 cup	no	4.0	56
puffed wheat	1 cup	no	3.7	44
GENERAL MILLS RAISIN BRAN	1 cup	no	3.2	178
KELLOGG'S RAISIN BRAN	1 cup	yes	3.1	186
RAISIN NUT BRAN	1 cup	no	3.8	209
REESE'S PEANUT BUTTER PUFFS	¾ cup	no	4.3	129
RICE KRISPIES	1 ¼ cup	no	3.8	124
RICE KRISPIES TREATS CEREAL	¾ cup	no	4.0	120
SHREDDED WHEAT	2 biscuits	yes	3.4	156
SMACKS	¾ cup	no	3.8	103
SPECIAL K	1 cup	no	3.7	115
QUAKER TOASTED OATMEAL	1 cup	no	3.9	191
TOTAL WHOLE GRAIN	¾ cup	no	3.5	105
TRIX	1 cup	no	4.1	122
WHEATIES	1 cup	no	3.7	110

Cake

Eating cake is not a good way to lose weight. Cake has a very high caloric density. Certain cakes should not be eaten at all (see table below). Some cakes, such as angel food cake, light yellow cake without frosting prepared from egg whites, and Boston cream pie, may be eaten occasionally. As you can see from the table below, these cakes are not as high in caloric density as other cakes are. Occasionally means a *small* piece once or twice a week.

Cake	Amount	Suggested Consumption	Caloric density (Cal/g)	Calories
angel food cake prepared from dry mix ($\frac{1}{12}$ of 10" diameter)	1 piece	occasionally	2.6	129
light yellow cake with water, egg whites, no frosting prepared from dry mix ($\frac{1}{12}$ of 9" diameter)	1 piece	occasionally	2.6	181
chocolate cake home-made without frosting ($\frac{1}{12}$ of 9" diameter)	1 piece	no	3.6	340
gingerbread home-made ($\frac{1}{9}$ of 8" square)	1 piece	no	3.6	263
pineapple upside-down cake home-made $\frac{1}{9}$ of 8" square	1 piece	no	3.2	367
shortcake home-made (3" dia)	1 shortcake	no	3.5	225
sponge cake home-made ($\frac{1}{12}$ of 16 oz cake)	1 piece	occasionally	3.0	187
white cake with coconut frosting home-made ($\frac{1}{12}$ of 9" diameter)	1 piece	no	3.6	399
white cake without frosting home-made ($\frac{1}{12}$ of 9" diameter)	1 piece	no	3.6	264
angel food cake commercially prepared ($\frac{1}{12}$ of 12 oz cake)	1 piece	occasionally	2.6	72
Boston cream pie commercially prepared ($\frac{1}{6}$ of pie)	1 piece	occasionally	2.5	232
chocolate cake with chocolate frosting, commercially prepared ($\frac{1}{8}$ of 18-oz cake)	1 piece	no	3.7	235
coffeecake commercially prepared ($\frac{1}{9}$ of 20 oz cake)	1 piece	no	4.2	263
fruitcake commercially prepared	1 piece	no	3.2	139
butter pound cake commercially prepared ($\frac{1}{12}$ of 12 oz cake)	1 piece	no	3.9	109

continued..

Cake	Amount	Suggested Consumption	Caloric density (Cal/g)	Calories
fat free pound cake (3 ¼" x 2 ¾" x ⅝" slice)	1 slice	occasionally	2.8	79
chocolate snack cake crème-filled, with frosting, commercially prepared	1 cupcake	no	3.8	188
chocolate snack cake with frosting low fat, commercially prepared	1 cupcake	no	3.1	131
sponge snack cake crème-filled, commercially prepared	1 cake	no	3.6	155
sponge cake commercially prepared	1 shortcake	occasionally	2.9	87
yellow cake with chocolate frosting, commercially prepared	1 piece	no	3.8	243
yellow cake with vanilla frosting, commercially prepared	1 piece	no	3.7	239
cheesecake (⅙ of 17 oz cake)	1 piece	no	3.2	257

Cookies, Crackers, and Muffins

Don't eat cookies, crackers, and muffins if you want to lose weight. They all have a high caloric density. Even cookies that are advertised as being lower in fat and calories have a high caloric density and should not be eaten. Instead have a fruit or a vegetable. A banana, some berries, melon, or maybe some yogurt, you get the idea.

Pasta and Noodles

You can eat pasta and noodles. Pasta and noodles have a low caloric density and can be safely eaten as part of a good weight-loss diet. Just don't eat huge portions!

Pie

Pie is fairly high in calories and saturated fat. Most pies have a lower caloric density than most cakes. Apple pie, blueberry pie, cherry pie, lemon meringue pie, and pumpkin pie can be eaten occasionally—a *small* piece once or twice a week. But if you eat pie twice a week, don't eat cake as well!

Pasta and Noodles	Amount	Suggested Consumption	Caloric density (Cal/g)	Calories
cooked macaroni	1 cup	yes	1.4	197
chow mein noodles	1 cup	no	5.3	237
cooked regular egg noodles	1 cup	yes	1.3	213
cooked spinach egg noodles	1 cup	yes	1.3	211
cooked spaghetti	1 cup	yes	1.4	197
cooked whole wheat spaghetti	1 cup	yes	1.2	174

Pie	Amount	Suggested Consumption	Caloric density (Cal/g)	Calories
standard pie crust*	1 pie shell	no	5.3	949
standard pie crust**	1 pie shell	no	5.1	648
graham cracker pie crust	1 pie shell	no	4.9	1181
apple pie**	1 piece	no	2.4	277
blueberry pie**	1 piece	occasionally	2.3	271
cherry pie**	1 piece	occasionally	2.6	304
chocolate crème pie**	1 piece	no	3.0	344
coconut custard pie**	1 piece	no	2.6	270
lemon meringue pie**	1 piece	occasionally	2.7	303
pecan pie**	1 piece	no	4.0	452
pumpkin pie**	1 piece	occasionally	2.1	229
apple pie*	1 piece	occasionally	2.7	411
blueberry pie*	1 piece	occasionally	2.5	360
cherry pie*	1 piece	occasionally	2.7	486
lemon meringue pie*	1 piece	occasionally	2.9	362
pecan pie*	1 piece	no	4.1	503
pumpkin pie*	1 piece	no	2.0	316
fried cherry pie	1 pie	no	3.2	404

*homemade   **commercially prepared

Snack Foods

Limit your snacks to 2 or 3 a day—1 between breakfast and lunch, 1 between lunch and dinner, and, if desired, 1 after dinner. If you learn only one thing from this book, it should be that it is important not to snack continuously throughout the day. Instead, eat three meals a day. Keep snack foods out of reach. Most of these foods have an extremely high caloric density. It is the continuous eating of high caloric density foods that is the cause of many cases of people becoming overweight and obese. If you get hungry during the day, have a piece of fruit (an apple or a banana), some vegetables (carrot sticks, celery sticks), a yogurt, or maybe nonfat pudding. It's alright to have a *few* nonfat potato chips.

Breakfast Foods Made from Grain

Most of these foods are high in calories, with a few exceptions. It is better to have fruit and low calorie cereal (e.g. cream of wheat or oatmeal) for breakfast than to fill up on bagels.

Breakfast Foods Made from Grain	Amount	Suggested Consumption	Caloric density (Cal/g)	Calories
plain bagel	4" bagel	avoid	2.8	245
cinnamon raisin bagel	4" bagel	in moderation	2.7	244
egg bagel	4" bagel	avoid	2.8	247
banana bread homemade prepared with margarine	1 slice	no	3.3	196
biscuits homemade prepared with 2% milk	4" biscuit	no	3.5	358
regular biscuits made from refrigerated dough	2½" biscuit	no	3.4	93
lower fat biscuits made from refrigerated dough	2¼" biscuit	no	3.0	63
breakfast bar, cereal crust, with fruit filling, fat free	1 bar	no	3.3	121
cornbread prepared from mix (3¾" x 2½" x ¾")	1 piece	no	3.1	188
cornbread homemade with 2% milk (2½" sq x 1½")	1 piece	avoid	2.7	173

continued..

Breakfast Foods Made from Grain	Amount	Suggested Consumption	Caloric density (Cal/g)	Calories
French toast homemade with 2% milk fried in margarine	1 slice	no	2.3	149
French toast frozen ready to heat	1 slice	yes	2.1	126
hard plain granola bar	1 bar	no	4.8	134
soft chocolate chip granola bar	1 bar	no	4.3	119
soft raisin granola bar	1 bar	no	4.5	127
soft chocolate-coated peanut butter granola bar	1 bar	no	5.1	144
NUTRI GRAIN cereal bar fruit filled	1 bar	no	3.7	136
frozen pancakes ready to heat (4" diameter)	1 pancake	in moderation	2.3	82
pancakes prepared from mix (4" diameter)	1 pancake	yes	2.0	74
cinnamon rolls with raisins	1 roll	no	3.7	223
refrigerated cinnamon rolls	1 roll	no	3.6	109
brown sugar cinnamon toaster pastries	1 pastry	no	4.1	206
chocolate toaster pastries with frosting	1 pastry	no	3.9	201
fruit filled toaster pastries	1 pastry	no	3.9	204
low fat toaster pastries	1 pastry	no	3.7	193
homemade waffles (7" diameter)	1 waffle	no	2.9	218
toasted frozen waffles (4" diameter)	1 waffle	avoid	2.6	87
low fat waffles (4" diameter)	1 waffle	in moderation	2.4	83

Rice and other grains

You can eat rice—it will help you lose weight.

Rice and Other Grains	Amount	Suggested Consumption	Caloric density (Cal/g)	Calories
barley cooked	1 cup	yes	1.2	193
buckwheat groats (kasha) cooked	1 cup	yes	0.9	155
bulgur cooked	1 cup	yes	0.8	151
couscous cooked	1 cup	yes	1.1	176
oat bran cooked	1 cup	yes	0.4	88
cooked brown rice	1 cup	yes	1.1	216
cooked white rice	1 cup	yes	1.3	205
prepared instant rice	1 cup	yes	1.0	162
cooked parboiled rice	1 cup	yes	1.1	200
cooked wild rice	1 cup	yes	1.0	166
rice cake	1 cake	no	3.9	350
tapioca	1 cup	no	3.6	544

Beans and Peas

Beans and peas are very healthy foods. They are low in calories and high in protein and fiber.

Beans and Peas	Amount	Suggested Consumption	Caloric density (Cal/g)	Calories
black beans	1 cup	yes	1.3	227
Great Northern beans	1 cup	yes	1.2	209
red kidney beans (dry)	1 cup	yes	1.3	225
lima beans (dry)	1 cup	yes	1.2	216
navy beans	1 cup	yes	1.4	258
pinto beans	1 cup	yes	1.4	234
vegetarian baked beans (canned)	1 cup	yes	0.9	236

continued..

Beans ans Peas	Amount	Suggested Consumption	Caloric density (Cal/g)	Calories
baked beans with frankfurters (canned)	1 cup	no	1.4	368
baked beans with pork in tomato sauce (canned)	1 cup	yes	1.0	248
baked beans with pork in sweet sauce (canned)	1 cup	yes	1.1	281
red kidney beans (canned)	1 cup	yes	0.9	218
lima beans (canned)	1 cup	yes	0.8	190
white beans (canned)	1 cup	yes	1.2	307
black eyed peas dry cooked	1 cup	yes	1.2	200
black eyed peas canned	1 cup	yes	0.8	185
chickpeas dry cooked	1 cup	yes	1.6	269
chickpeas canned	1 cup	yes	1.2	286
hummus	1 tbsp	yes	1.6	23
lentils cooked	1 cup	yes	1.2	230
peas cooked	1 cup	yes	1.2	231
refried beans canned	1 cup	yes	0.9	237
soybeans cooked	1 cup	yes	1.7	298
miso	1 cup	in moderation	2.1	567
soy milk	1 cup	in moderation	0.3	81
tofu firm	¼ block	yes	0.8	62
tofu soft piece	1 piece	yes	0.6	73

Nuts, Seeds, and Peanuts

Nuts and peanuts have been shown to protect against heart disease. Eat 5–10 ounces a week. Peanut butter—if it has added partially hydrogenated oil—does not have the same protective effect against heart disease. However natural peanut butter—made just from peanuts—probably has the same protective effect. Understand that nuts and peanuts have a high caloric density and will cause you to gain weight if you eat too many.

Nuts, Seeds, and Peanuts	Amount	Suggested Consumption	Caloric density (Cal/g)	Calories
almonds, shelled, whole	1 oz	yes	5.9	164
Brazil nuts (6-8 nuts)	1 oz	yes	6.6	186
cashews, dry roasted	1 oz	yes	5.8	163
cashews, oil roasted (18 nuts)	1 oz	yes	5.8	163
chestnuts, shelled	1 cup	yes	2.5	350
coconut, raw, piece	1 piece	no	3.5	159
coconut, raw, shredded	1 cup	no	3.5	283
coconut, dried	1 cup	no	5.0	466
hazelnuts, chopped	1 oz	yes	6.4	178
macadamia nuts, salted (10-12 nuts)	1 oz	yes	7.3	203
mixed nuts with peanuts, salted, dry roasted	1 oz	yes	6.0	168
mixed nuts with peanuts, salted, oil roasted	1 oz	in moderation	6.3	175
pecans (20 halves)	1 oz	yes	7.0	196
pine nuts, shelled	1 oz	yes	5.7	160
pistachio nuts, salted, shelled (47 nuts)	1 oz	yes	5.8	161
pumpkin and squash seeds, salted (142 seeds)	1 oz	yes	5.3	148
sesame seeds	1 tbsp	yes	5.9	47
tahini	1 tbsp	yes	5.9	89
sunflower seeds, roasted with salt	1 oz	yes	5.9	165
walnuts (14 halves)	1 oz	yes	6.6	185
peanuts, salted, dry roasted (about 28)	1 oz	yes	5.9	166
peanuts, unsalted, dry roasted (about 28)	1 oz	yes	5.9	166
peanuts, salted, oil roasted	1 cup	yes	5.8	837
peanut butter, regular, smooth	1 tbsp	no	5.9	95
peanut butter, regular, chunky	1 tbsp	no	5.9	94
peanut butter, reduced fat, smooth	1 tbsp	no	5.2	94

Meat and Meat Products

Beef: don't eat it for dinner. Don't eat it for breakfast or lunch either. Unfortunately, beef, pork, and lamb are high in saturated fat. Eating meat will increase your risk of heart disease. My advice: don't.

It's alright to have a portion of eye of round roast from which the fat has been cut away (caloric density 1.7)* or braised veal cutlet (caloric density 2.1)† *occasionally*. By occasionally, I mean once a week.

I understand that many people will be unwilling to completely cut out other red meats from their diets. In addition to eye of round roast and braised veal cutlet, several other meats will not cause you to gain weight. These include sirloin steak, roast lamb leg, roast ham, and Canadian bacon—but be sure to cut away the fat. I cannot really recommend these 4 foods since they have a fair amount of saturated animal fat that could increase your risk of heart disease, but at least they are not as high in saturated fats as some other meats.

Mixed Dishes and Fast Foods

Most mixed dishes, fast foods, and prepared foods are unhealthy because they contain a large amount of saturated fat, and eating a large amount of saturated fat increases the risk of heart disease. In general, it would be better not to eat fast food. Note that there are a few prepared foods, such as some of the Healthy Choice® and Morningstar Farms® products, that are both healthy to eat and low in calories.

It's alright to eat a tuna sandwich. Mashed potatoes are good to eat—particularly if they are made without milk or with skim milk. Some other foods you may be surprised to learn are fine to have *occasionally* (once a week, small portion): pizza with vegetables or a roast beef sandwich.

Mixed Dishes and Fast Foods	Amount	Suggested Consumption	Caloric density (Cal/g)	Calories
HEALTHY CHOICE® beef macaroni	1 package	yes	0.9	211
canned beef stew	1 cup	no	0.9	218
chicken pot pie	1 small pie	no	2.2	484
chili con carne with beans canned	1 cup	yes	1.2	255
macaroni and cheese canned	1 cup	no	0.8	199

continued..

* Six ounces of eye of round roast from which the fat has been cut away has 286 calories.
† Six ounces of braised veal cutlet has 358 calories

Mixed Dishes and Fast Foods	Amount	Suggested Consumption	Caloric density (Cal/g)	Calories
MORNINGSTAR FARMS® meatless burger crumbles	1 cup	no	2.1	231
MORNINGSTAR FARMS® meatless burger patty	1 patty	yes	1.1	91
pasta with meatballs in tomato sauce, canned	1 cup	no	1.0	260
HEALTHY CHOICE® spaghetti Bolognese	1 package	yes	0.9	255
spaghetti in tomato sauce with cheese canned	1 cup	yes	0.8	192
spinach souffle	1 cup	no	1.6	219
cheese tortellini frozen	¾ cup	no	3.1	249
biscuit with egg and sausage	1 biscuit	no	3.2	581
croissant with egg, cheese, bacon	1 croissant	no	3.2	413
cheese danish	1 pastry	no	3.9	353
fruit danish	1 pastry	no	3.6	335
English muffin with egg, cheese, Canadian bacon	1 muffin	no	2.1	289
French toast with butter	2 slices	no	2.6	356
French toast sticks	5 sticks	no	3.6	513
hash brown potatoes	½ cup	no	2.1	151
pancakes with butter, syrup	2 pancakes	no	2.2	520
bean and cheese burrito	1 burrito	no	2.0	189
bean and meat burrito	1 burrito	no	2.2	255
cheeseburger double patty with mayo type dressing, vegetables	1 sandwich	no	2.5	417
cheeseburger single patty with mayo type dressing, vegetables	1 sandwich	no	2.6	295
cheeseburger double patty	1 sandwich	no	3.0	457
cheeseburger double patty with 3 piece bun	1 sandwich	no	2.9	461
cheeseburger single patty	1 sandwich	no	3.1	319
large cheeseburger single patty with mayo type dressing, vegetables	1 sandwich	no	2.6	563
large cheeseburger single patty with bacon	1 sandwich	no	3.1	608
chicken fillet breaded and fried sandwich	1 sandwich	no	2.8	515

continued..

Mixed Dishes and Fast Foods	Amount	Suggested Consumption	Caloric density (Cal/g)	Calories
boneless chicken pieces breaded and fried	6 pieces	no	3.0	319
chili con carne	1 cup	no	1.0	256
chimichanga with beef	1	no	2.4	425
coleslaw	¾ cup	in moderation	1.5	147
ice milk vanilla desert in cone	1 cone	no	1.6	164
fried pie with fruit filling	1 pie	no	3.2	404
hot fudge sundae	1 sundae	no	1.8	284
enchilada with cheese	1 enchilada	no	2.0	319
fish sandwich with tartar sauce and cheese	1 sandwich	no	2.9	523
french fries	1 small	no	3.4	291
french fries	1 medium	no	3.4	458
french fries	1 large	no	3.4	578
frijoles	1 cup	yes	1.4	225
hamburger regular size with condiments double patty	1 sandwich	no	2.7	576
hamburger regular size with condiments single patty	1 sandwich	no	2.6	272
hamburger large double patty with condiments mayo type dressing and vegetables	1 sandwich	no	2.4	540
hamburger large single patty with condiments mayo type dressing and vegetables	1 sandwich	no	2.4	512
hot dog plain	1 sandwich	no	2.5	242
hot dog with chili	1 sandwich	no	2.6	296
corndog	1 corndog	occasionally	2.6	460
hush puppies	5 pieces	no	3.3	257
mashed potatoes	⅓ cup	yes	0.8	66
nachos with cheese sauce	6-8 nachos	no	3.1	346
onion rings breaded and fried	8-9 rings	no	3.3	276
cheese pizza	1 slice	occasionally	2.2	140
pizza with meat and vegetables	1 slice	occasionally	2.3	184
pepperoni pizza	1 slice	no	2.6	181
roast beef sandwich	1 sandwich	occasionally	2.5	346
tossed salad with chicken no dressing	1½ cups	yes	0.5	105
tossed salad with egg, cheese, no dressing	1½ cups	no	0.5	102

continued..

Mixed Dishes and Fast Foods	Amount	Suggested Consumption	Caloric density (Cal/g)	Calories
chocolate shake	16 fl oz	no	1.3	423
vanilla shake	16 fl oz	no	1.1	370
breaded fried shrimp	6-8 shrimp	no	2.8	454
submarine sandwich with cold cuts	1 sandwich	no	2.0	456
submarine sandwich with roast beef	1 sandwich	no	1.9	410
submarine sandwich with tuna salad	1 sandwich	in moderation	2.9	584
beef taco	1 large	no	2.2	568
taco salad (ground beef, cheese, taco shell)	1 ½ cups	no	1.4	279
tostada with beans and beef	1 tostada	no	1.5	333

Poultry

Chicken and turkey can be a healthy part of the diet and a good source of protein. The trick is to remove the skin, which contains most of the fat. Also, chicken and turkey breast light meat have less saturated fat than dark meat. Needless to say, frying chicken increases the amount of saturated fat and the number of calories.

Poultry	Amount	Suggested Consumption	Caloric density (Cal/g)	Calories
fried chicken breast	½ breast	no	2.6	364
fried chicken drumstick	1 drumstick	no	2.7	193
fried chicken thigh	1 thigh	no	2.8	238
fried chicken wing	1 wing	no	3.2	159
roasted chicken breast without skin	½ breast	yes	1.7	142
roasted chicken drumstick without skin	1 drumstick	in moderation	1.7	76

continued..

Poultry	Amount	Suggested Consumption	Caloric density (Cal/g)	Calories
roasted chicken thigh without skin	1 thigh	no	2.1	109
roasted chicken breast with skin	½ breast	in moderation	2.0	193
roasted chicken drumstick with skin	1 drumstick	no	2.2	112
roasted chicken thigh with skin	1 thigh	no	2.5	153
stewed chicken	1 cup	no	2.4	332
chicken giblets simmered	1 cup	no	1.6	228
chicken liver simmered	1 liver	no	1.6	31
chicken neck simmered	1 neck	no	1.8	32
roast duck	½ duck	no	2.0	444
roast turkey dark meat and skin	6 oz	no	2.2	376
roast turkey light meat and skin	6 oz	no	2.0	334
roast turkey dark meat without skin	6 oz	no	1.9	318
roast turkey light meat without skin	6 oz	yes	1.6	266
cooked ground turkey patty	1 patty	no	2.4	193
turkey giblets simmered	1 cup	no	1.7	242
turkey neck simmered	1 neck	no	1.8	274
canned chicken	5 oz	no	1.6	234
chicken frankfurter	1 frank	no	2.6	116
light meat chicken roll	2 slices	no	1.6	90
turkey patties breaded fried	1 patty	no	2.8	181

Soup

Soup is low in calories and is a good way to fill you up without taking in too many calories. If you have high blood pressure that is "salt-sensitive," be aware that many soups are high in sodium.

Soup	Amount	Suggested Consumption	Caloric density (Cal/g)	Calories
New England clam chowder	1 cup	no	0.7	164
cream of chicken	1 cup	no	0.8	191
cream of mushroom	1 cup	no	0.8	203
cream of tomato	1 cup	no	0.7	161
bean with pork	1 cup	in moderation	0.7	172
beef bouillon	1 cup	yes	0.1	29
beef noodle	1 cup	in moderation	0.3	83
chicken noodle	1 cup	yes	0.3	75
chicken and rice	1 cup	yes	0.3	60
Manhattan clam chowder	1 cup	yes	0.3	78
cream of chicken	1 cup	no	0.5	117
cream of mushroom	1 cup	no	0.5	129
minestrone	1 cup	yes	0.3	82
pea	1 cup	yes	0.7	165
tomato	1 cup	yes	0.4	85
vegetable beef	1 cup	in moderation	0.3	78
vegetable	1 cup	yes	0.3	72
chunky bean with ham	1 cup	no	1.0	231
chunky chicken noodle	1 cup	yes	0.7	175
chunky chicken vegetable	1 cup	yes	0.7	166
vegetable	1 cup	yes	0.5	122
chicken broth★	1 cup	yes	0.1	17
chicken noodle, low fat★	1 cup	yes	0.3	76
chicken and rice, low fat★	1 cup	yes	0.5	116
chicken and rice with vegetables★	1 cup	yes	0.4	88
New England clam chowder, low fat★	1 cup	yes	0.5	117
lentil soup, reduced sodium	1 cup	yes	0.5	126
minestrone soup★	1 cup	yes	0.5	123
vegetable soup★	1 cup	yes	0.3	81
beef soup, homemade	1 cup	yes	0.3	31
chicken soup, homemade	1 cup	yes	0.9	86
fish soup, homemade	1 cup	yes	0.4	40

★ reduced sodium

Sauces and gravies

It is alright to use sauces and gravies to flavor your foods. Avoid sauces such as cheese sauce that are high in saturated fat. Most sauces are high in sodium, so be careful if you have "salt-sensitive" high blood pressure.

Sauces and Gravies	Amount	Suggested Consumption	Caloric density (Cal/g)	Calories
cheese sauce, homemade	1 cup	no	2.0	479
white sauce, homemade with milk	1 cup	no	1.5	368
barbecue sauce	1 tbsp	in moderation	0.8	12
cheese sauce	¼ cup	no	1.8	110
hoisin sauce	1 tbsp	yes	2.2	35
nacho cheese sauce	¼ cup	no	1.9	119
pepper or hot sauce	1 tsp	yes	0.2	1
salsa	1 tbsp	yes	0.3	4
soy sauce	1 tbsp	yes	0.6	9
marinara sauce	1 cup	yes	0.6	143
teriyaki sauce	1 tbsp	no	0.8	15
tomato chili sauce	¼ cup	yes	1.0	71
Worcestershire sauce	1 tbsp	yes	0.7	11
beef gravy	¼ cup	in moderation	0.5	31
chicken gravy	¼ cup	yes	0.8	47
country sausage gravy	¼ cup	no	1.6	96
mushroom gravy	¼ cup	yes	0.5	30
turkey gravy	¼ cup	yes	0.5	31

Candy

Don't eat candy if you want to lose weight. Candy has a high caloric density. Most candy is also high in saturated fat. If you must have candy, limit the amount that you eat.

Other sweets

Other sweets can be a good alternative to candy. You can have some frozen ices. Jello is also good—and reduced-calorie jello made with NutraSweet has almost no calories. You may use some jam or jelly, just limit your consumption of these—they have fairly high caloric densities.

Other Sweets	Amount	Suggested Consumption	Caloric density (Cal/g)	Calories
chocolate frosting	1/12 package	no	4.0	151
vanilla frosting	1/12 package	no	4.2	159
frozen fruit bar	1 bar	in moderation	0.8	63
ice pop	1 bar	in moderation	0.7	42
Italian ices	1/2 cup	yes	0.5	61
apple butter	1 tbsp	yes	1.7	29
regular gelatin	1/2 cup	yes	0.6	80
reduced calorie gelatin with aspartame	1/2 cup	yes	0.1	8
honey	1 tbsp	no	3.1	64
jams and preserves	1 tbsp	in moderation	2.8	56
jellies	1 tbsp	in moderation	2.8	54

Puddings

Pudding is a nice sweet treat that you can eat—it is healthy and low in calories. In particular, nonfat pudding is very healthy and has a very low caloric density.

Puddings	Amount	Suggested Consumption	Caloric density (Cal/g)	Calories
chocolate pudding★	1/2 cup	in moderation	1.0	150
chocolate pudding★★	1/2 cup	in moderation	1.1	151
vanilla pudding★	1/2 cup	in moderation	1.0	148
vanilla pudding★★	1/2 cup	in moderation	1.0	141
chocolate pudding★★★	1/2 cup	yes	1.3	150
rice pudding★★★	1/2 cup	in moderation	1.6	184
tapioca pudding★★★	1/2 cup	yes	1.2	134

continued..

Puddings	Amount	Suggested Consumption	Caloric density (Cal/g)	Calories
vanilla pudding★★★	½ cup	yes	1.3	147
chocolate pudding, fat free★★★	½ cup	Yes	1.0	107
tapioca pudding, fat free★★★	½ cup	Yes	0.9	98
vanilla pudding, fat free★★★	½ cup	Yes	0.9	105

★ prepared from dry mix instant

★★ prepared from dry mix cooked

★★★ regular ready to eat

Sugar

Sugar has a very high caloric density. Reducing the amount of sugar you are eating will reduce the number of calories you are taking in.

Syrup

Syrups are high in calories and should be used sparingly. Reduced calorie syrup is better.

Syrup	Amount	Suggested Consumption	Caloric density (Cal/g)	Calories
chocolate syrup	1 tbsp	sparingly	2.8	53
chocolate fudge syrup	1 tbsp	no	3.5	67
light corn syrup	1 tbsp	sparingly	2.8	56
maple syrup	1 tbsp	sparingly	2.6	52
molasses	1 tbsp	sparingly	2.4	47
regular pancake syrup	1 tbsp	sparingly	2.9	57
reduced calorie pancake syrup	1 tbsp	yes	1.7	25

Vegetables

Eating vegetables is an excellent way to lose weight. You should try to have 4 servings or more a day. What counts as a serving? 1 cup of raw leafy vegetables, ½ cup of other vegetables, or ¾ cup of vegetable juice.

Vegetables	Amount	Suggested Consumption	Caloric density (Cal/g)	Calories
alfalfa sprouts	1 cup	yes	0.3	10
artichokes	1 medium	yes	0.5	60
asparagus	4 spears	yes	0.2	14
bamboo shoots	1 cup	yes	0.2	25
beets	1 beet	yes	0.4	22
beet greens	1 cup	yes	0.3	39
broccoli	1 cup	yes	0.3	25
brussels sprouts	1 cup	yes	0.4	65
cabbage	1 cup	yes	0.3	18
Chinese cabbage (bok choy)	1 cup	yes	0.1	20
carrot juice	1 cup	yes	0.4	94
carrots	1 carrot	yes	0.4	31
baby carrots	1 medium	yes	0.4	4
cauliflower	1 floweret	yes	0.2	3
celery	1 stalk	yes	0.2	6
chives	1 tbsp	yes	0.3	1
cilantro	1 tsp	yes	0.0	0
coleslaw	1 cup	yes	0.7	83
collards	1 cup	yes	0.4	61
corn on the cob	1 ear	yes	1.1	83
creamed corn	1 cup	yes	0.7	184
white sweet corn	1 ear	yes	1.1	83
cucumber	1 large	yes	0.1	39
dandelion greens	1 cup	yes	0.3	35
dill weed	5 sprigs	yes	0.0	0
eggplant	1 cup	yes	0.3	28
endive	1 cup	yes	0.2	9
garlic	1 clove	yes	1.3	4
hearts of palm	1 piece	yes	0.3	9

continued..

Vegetables	Amount	Suggested Consumption	Caloric density (Cal/g)	Calories
Jerusalem artichoke	1 cup	yes	0.8	114
kale	1 cup	yes	0.3	39
kohlrabi	1 cup	yes	0.3	48
leeks	1 cup	yes	0.3	32
lettuce head, butterhead	1 head	yes	0.1	21
lettuce, iceberg	1 cup	yes	0.1	7
lettuce, looseleaf	1 cup	yes	0.2	10
lettuce, romaine	1 cup	yes	0.1	8
mushrooms	1 cup	yes	0.3	18
mushrooms, shiitake, cooked	1 cup	yes	0.6	80
mushrooms, shiitake, dried	1 mushroom	in moderation	2.8	11
mustard greens	1 cup	yes	0.2	21
okra, cooked	1 cup	yes	0.3	52
onions	1 whole	yes	0.4	42
onion rings	10 rings	no	4.1	244
parsley	10 sprigs	yes	0.4	4
parsnips	1 cup	yes	0.8	126
green hot chili peppers	1 pepper	yes	0.4	18
red hot chili peppers	1 pepper	yes	0.4	18
jalapeno peppers	¼ cup	yes	0.3	7
sweet green peppers	1 pepper	yes	0.3	32
sweet red peppers	1 pepper	yes	0.3	32
pimento	1 tbsp	yes	0.3	3
baked potato, flesh only	1 potato	yes	0.9	145
baked potato, skin only	1 skin	yes	2.0	115
boiled potatoes, peeled	1 potato	yes	0.9	116
potato au gratin, from dry mix, with whole milk, butter	1 cup	no	0.9	228
potato au gratin, homemade, with butter	1 cup	no	1.3	323
French fried potatoes, frozen, heated	10 strips	yes	2.0	100
hashed brown potatoes	1 patty	no	2.2	63
mashed potatoes from flakes with whole milk, butter, and salt	1 cup	no	1.1	237
mashed potatoes, homemade with whole milk	1 cup	yes	0.8	162

continued..

Vegetables	Amount	Suggested Consumption	Caloric density (Cal/g)	Calories
homemade mashed potatoes with whole milk and margarine	1 cup	in moderation	1.1	223
potato pancakes	1 pancake	no	2.7	207
potato puffs	10 puffs	no	2.2	175
potato salad	1 cup	in moderation	1.4	358
scalloped potatoes	1 cup	no	0.9	211
pumpkin	1 cup	yes	0.2	49
radishes	1 radish	yes	0.2	1
rutabagas	1 cup	yes	0.4	66
sauerkraut	1 cup	in moderation	0.2	45
seaweed, kelp	2 tbsp	yes	0.4	4
seaweed, spirulina	1 tbsp	no	3.0	3
shallots	1 tbsp	yes	0.7	7
raw leaf spinach	1 leaf	yes	0.2	2
spinach, cooked	1 cup	yes	0.3	53
summer squash	1 cup	yes	0.2	36
winter squash	1 cup	yes	0.4	80
butternut squash, cooked, mashed	1 cup	yes	0.4	94
baked sweet potatoes with skin	1 potato	yes	1.0	150
boiled sweet potatoes without skin	1 potato	yes	1.1	164
candied sweet potatoes	1 piece	in moderation	1.4	144
canned sweet potatoes, packed in syrup	1 cup	yes	1.1	212
tomatillos	1 medium	yes	0.3	11
cherry tomatoes	1 cherry	yes	0.2	4
medium tomatoes	1 tomato	yes	0.2	26
canned tomatoes	1 cup	yes	0.2	46
sun dried tomatoes, plain	1 piece	yes	2.5	5
sun dried tomatoes, packed in oil	1 piece	yes	2.0	6
tomato juice	1 cup	yes	0.2	41
tomato paste	1 cup	yes	0.8	215
tomato puree	1 cup	yes	0.4	100
tomato sauce	1 cup	yes	0.3	74
stewed tomatoes	1 cup	yes	0.3	71

continued..

Vegetables	Amount	Suggested Consumption	Caloric density (Cal/g)	Calories
turnips	1 cup	yes	0.2	33
turnip greens	1 cup	yes	0.2	29
vegetable juice cocktail	1 cup	yes	0.2	46
canned mixed vegetables	1 cup	yes	0.5	77
frozen mixed vegetables	1 cup	yes	0.6	107
water chestnuts	1 cup	yes	0.5	70

Condiments

Feel free to use condiments to flavor your food. If you have "salt-sensitive" high blood pressure, be aware that ketchup and mustard have a fair amount of sodium.

Condiments	Amount	Suggested Consumption	Caloric density (Cal/g)	Calories
ketchup	1 tbsp	yes	1.1	16
horseradish	1 tsp	yes	0.4	2
mustard	1 tsp	yes	0.6	3
pickle relish	1 tbsp	yes	1.3	20

Olives and Pickles

Olives and pickles are good to eat. If you have "salt-sensitive" high blood pressure, be aware they can have a lot of sodium.

Olives and Pickles	Amount	Suggested Consumption	Caloric density (Cal/g)	Calories
green olives	5 medium	yes	1.2	20
black olives	5 large	yes	1.1	25
dill pickles	1 pickle	yes	0.2	12
fresh pickles	3 slices	yes	0.8	18

Spices

Spices are a good way to flavor your food. Feel free to use them. Adding spices can make bland food taste better.

Food	Amount	Suggested Consumption	Caloric density (Cal/g)	Calories
chili powder	1 tsp	yes	2.7	8
cinnamon	1 tsp	yes	3.0	6
curry powder	1 tsp	yes	3.5	7
garlic powder	1 tsp	yes	3.0	9
onion powder	1 tsp	yes	3.5	7
oregano	1 tsp	yes	2.5	5
paprika	1 tsp	yes	3.0	6
dried parsley	1 tbsp	yes	4.0	4
black pepper	1 tsp	yes	2.5	5
vanilla extract	1 tsp	yes	3.0	12

Salt

You can have salt, just don't overdo it, particularly if you have "salt-sensitive" high blood pressure. Pepper is fine.

Chapter 10

EXERCISE

Exercise Improves Health in Several Ways

First, people who are dieting who also exercise will lose more weight.[269] The more calories you burn, the more weight you will lose (assuming you don't eat more!) Whether exercising intensely will help you lose more weight than exercising moderately is still debated by physicians.[270] Does exercise increase your appetite? We really don't know. However, we do know for certain that if you exercise in addition to dieting you will lose more weight than if you don't exercise.

Second, exercise helps prevent heart disease and conditions the body to withstand serious disease in general.[271] A study of 17,944 British civil servants found that exercise cut the risk of developing heart disease in half.[272] A study of 17,321 Harvard alumni confirmed the benefits of exercise.[273] Since these classic studies, there have been many studies confirming the benefits of exercise in reducing the risk of heart disease.

I recommend you start off doing 30 minutes a day of moderate physical activity. An example of moderate physical activity would be a brisk walk (i.e. a 15 minute mile pace).

As your body gets conditioned, gradually increase the amount of time you are exercising to 60 minutes a day. And gradually increase the intensity of your exercise.

If you are able to exercise 90 minutes a day, this will be even more effective in helping you lose weight. 90 minutes may sound extreme, and I realize not all people are willing or have the time to exercise that much. You should be aware though that the scientific data indicates that 60-90 minutes of exercise a day is more effective in preventing weight gain than 30 minutes of exercise a day.[274]

If you can't do 90 minutes, then do 60. If you can't do 60, do 30. Let me be clear though. This book is for people who really want to lose weight. It is certainly very possible to lose weight without exercising by eating low caloric density foods. There is no question though, that if you are committed to losing weight and are willing to exercise 60 to 90 minutes a day and also eat low caloric density foods, this will make losing weight much easier.

Exercise is not just for young adults! I have had older patients say to me, "I'm too old to exercise." However, the scientific literature is clear. If you are over 65 or even over 75, you will lower your chance of a heart attack and will extend your life by exercising.[275,276]

Children should participate in at least 60 minutes of moderate physical activity daily. In fact 60 minutes should be the bare minimum for children—at least 90 minutes would be better.

Before becoming more physically active, certain people need to talk with their doctors. This includes people with chronic health problems such as heart disease, high blood pressure, diabetes, osteoporosis, and obesity; people with risk factors for heart disease (people with a family history of heart disease and cigarette smokers); and men over 40 and women over 50.

This does not mean that people with heart disease should not exercise! Exercise will help people with heart disease lose weight. It will slow the progression of or even reverse heart disease. And it has been shown that people with heart disease who adopt a regular exercise program have a lower death rate and live longer.[277] People with heart disease just need some supervision of intensity and duration so they don't have a heart attack—it is especially important for people with heart disease to build up their exercise level gradually.

The more vigorous the activity, the faster you burn calories. Below is a table of different exercises listing how many calories you burn in an hour.[278]

Activity	Your Weight		
	100 lb	150 lb	200 lb
bicycling, 6 mph	160	240	312
bicycling, 12 mph	270	410	534
jogging, 8:30 minute mile pace	610	920	1230
jumping, rope	500	750	1000
running, 11 minute mile pace	440	660	962
running, 6 minute mile pace	850	1280	1664
swimming, 25 yds/min	185	275	358
swimming, 50 yds/min	325	500	650
tennis	265	400	535
walking, 30 minute mile pace	160	240	312
walking, 20 minute mile pace	210	320	416
walking, 13:20 minute mile pace	295	440	572

Chapter 11

How Fast to Lose Weight

Women should start off with a 1000–1200 calorie/day diet.[279] Men should start off with a 1200–1600 calorie/day diet. Women over 165 pounds or who exercise regularly may also start off with a 1200–1600 calorie/day diet. If you are losing weight but are hungry, increase your caloric intake by 100–200 calories a day. In no case should you consume fewer than 800 calories a day—you need at least 800 calories a day to stay healthy and prevent muscle breakdown.

You should lose 1–2 pounds a week. Don't lose more than 2 pounds a weeks—it isn't healthy. For example, people who lose weight too fast can get gallstone disease.

If you are overweight but not obese (BMI 25–29.9), you may lose ½ pound a week. People who are overweight but not obese do not need to lose weight as quickly as obese people.

If you are not losing weight or are losing less than 1 pound a week, decrease the number of calories you are consuming. You can decrease the number of calories you are consuming by either decreasing the amount of food you are eating or by avoiding foods with a caloric density greater than 2.

If you are losing more than 2 pounds a week, increase the number of calories you are consuming. You can do this by either increasing the amount of food you are eating or by eating some foods with a caloric density between 2 and 3.

Of course, you should weigh yourself at least once a week so that you can adjust the amount of calories you are consuming appropriately.

Your initial goal should be to lose about 10% of your body weight in 6 months to a year. For example if you weigh 200 pounds in January, your goal should be to weigh 180 pounds in July.

Once you reach a normal BMI (that is, a BMI of 18.5-24.9), *gradually* increase the number of calories you are consuming until your weight stabilizes.

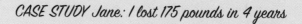

CASE STUDY Jane: I lost 175 pounds in 4 years

I came from a family that ate fattening foods. When I was 22 I weighed 300 pounds.

When I got to medical school I spent a lot of time reading about different diets because I was intent on losing weight.

I read about the low fat diets and about the low carb diets. None of them were based on scientific knowledge, and I decided not to follow any of them. I happened upon the right diet—the Golden Gate Diet—and I decided that it would be the diet I would follow.

I always eat 3 meals a day and 2 snacks. I use the caloric density charts to determine which foods I can safely eat. I limit sweets to an occasional piece of candy, and I cook with sugar-free sweeteners.

I walk at least 45 minutes every day, and I do some weight training. My efforts have paid off.

It's taken 4 years, but I've lost 175 pounds, and I feel wonderful. I no longer feel self-conscious. I have now started to date.

The Golden Gate Diet has given me a new lease on life, and I am now looking forward to starting a residency program. As part of the program I intend to do research on eating problems.

Chapter 12

ONCE YOU LOSE WEIGHT, KEEP IT OFF

Once you achieve your weight loss goal, you can't stop the diet or you will gain back the weight you lost! **The changes in diet and exercise you make need to be life-long changes.** Of course, you will be following a weight maintenance diet rather than a weight loss diet. You will be able to eat more calories since at this point you will need only to burn as many calories as you consume. (When you want to lose weight, as opposed to maintain weight, you need to burn *more* calories than you consume.)

You will see it's not at all hard to do.

Everyone will have days when they "slip up" and fail to stick to the diet. That's OK. When that happens, don't dwell on it, just go back on the diet the next day.

As you begin to lose weight, you will notice you start feeling better about your body. Your self-esteem will improve. This is in turn will make it easier to stick to the diet and keep a low weight over the long-term.

Get Support From your Family, Friends, and Doctor

Encouragement to lose weight and to stick to your diet from your family and friends will make your sticking with the diet much easier. Your family and friends can help you!

If you have health problems or are obese (BMI greater than 30) talk with your doctor. He or she can help you with the diet and help you stick to it! He or she can make sure your diet is going safely.

CASE STUDY Lillian: Social success

I've had a problem with food since I was a child. When I went to school the kids would call me "fatso", and that made me feel terrible. My mother tried to help by preparing foods that were low in calories, but I have a sweet tooth. When Mom wasn't looking I would eat candy bars.

For 35 years I tried one diet or another. I even tried to go without food for a few days. Unfortunately, I always went off the diet and gained all the weight back. I felt self-conscious and was unable to establish a committed relationship.

I threw myself into my work and became a workaholic. Though I had little hope of losing weight, I was introduced to the Golden Gate Diet.

On the Golden Gate Diet, I've lost 30 pounds, and I am now normal weight.

I can't tell you how happy I am. For the first time in my life I've lost weight and am able to keep the weight off without too much difficulty. As I said, a problem I have is I love sweets. I have to make sure that I don't have any at home, so I won't be tempted to eat sweets when I'm tired. Aside from avoiding sweets, it isn't hard to follow the diet. It doesn't take long to prepare the food. I am never hungry.

On the Golden Gate Diet I choose to eat mainly fish, chicken, turkey, vegetables, fruit, potatoes, and rice. I also eat yogurt, which gives me extra calcium. I found that on the Golden Gate Diet, you can make substitutions. You don't have to follow the meal plans exactly—if I don't want to eat chicken one day, I can eat fish instead. When I substitute, I try to substitute foods with roughly the same numbers of calories.

I've gotten a new wardrobe, thrown out my old clothes, and I am so pleased with the way I look and feel.

Because I feel less insecure, I spend less time at work, and I have developed a lot more friendships—I have a lot more friends than I did before.

Eating out

Eating a healthy diet in a restaurant can be a challenge—but with a little thought, it can be done. Try to stick to foods that are low in caloric density and low in saturated fat.

The portion sizes in American restaurants are huge. If you go to France, for example, restaurants serve much smaller portions. The bottom line is that American restaurants give you more food than most people need. **Do not** feel obligated to eat all the food they give you in a restaurant. It's usually a good idea to leave food over.

Limit alcoholic drinks—maybe have just one glass of wine. Avoid regular soda—have diet soda or water instead. Skip the bread and rolls. Have some soup—just avoid cream-based soups. Have some salad and go easy on the dressing. Avoid red meat dishes. Have fish instead. Or have chicken—just ask the chef to remove the skin. Avoid fried foods—have baked, broiled, or grilled foods instead. Have some pasta or rice. Avoid dishes with cheese and ask the chef to make your dinner without cheese. Eat plenty of vegetables. For dessert, have pie or mixed fruit. Skip the ice cream and cake.

Part of the problem is that when people go out to a restaurant they are very hungry when they get there. What is the first thing you are served? Bread and butter, which have a high caloric density. To avoid filling up on bread and butter, consider having a low caloric density snack, such as a piece of fruit, a salad, or the like, before you go out.

Chapter 13

A Psychology of Overeating

Overeating can be divided into 2 categories:

Taking in too many calories when you are hungry.

Taking in calories when you are not hungry.

What's great about the Golden Gate Diet is that it satisfies your appetite and makes you feel not hungry without giving you a lot of calories—by telling you to eat foods with a low caloric density.

When will this not work?

1. If you eat high caloric density food.

2. If you eat when you are not hungry.

Why do people eat high caloric density food or eat when they are not hungry? These are problems of the mind.

The truth is that doctors do not fully understand why people eat foods that will cause them to gain weight or why people eat when they are not hungry. We do understand some things, though.

Self-efficacy

"Self-efficacy" means that one has the belief that one will succeed.

If you are overweight and believe you will succeed at losing weight and keeping the weight off, you have a good chance of success.[280]

If you are overweight and do not believe you will succeed at losing weight, you have a poor chance of success.

It's important to know that if you "slip up" one day and eat high caloric density food, it's not the end of the world. Don't give up! Go back on the Golden Gate Diet. One day's not going to kill your diet. Just remember, the fewer days you "slip up", the faster you are going to lose weight.

Control

"Control" means that one has the ability to control one's behavior. When people get "out of control", they may eat a lot or eat the wrong foods when they do not feel hungry. They may feel they are unable to stop themselves.[281]

Stress

Some people eat in response to stress.[282] When they feel anxious, they eat as a way to relieve their anxiety. This can lead to a lot of eating when one is not hungry—and a lot of extra calories. What's worse, people who eat in response to stress often eat high caloric density foods.

Depression

Many people eat when they feel depressed.[283] Eating when you are not hungry and eating high caloric density foods will lead to weight gain. Becoming overweight and obese can cause depression.[284] A vicious cycle is created.

What can be done?

When there is a psychological cause of being overweight, a psychological treatment is needed.

The quickest way is through behavioral therapy, which is discussed in chapter 15. A trained mental health professional, such as a psychiatrist, psychologist, social worker or other trained mental health professional, can help you change your behaviors so that you can make healthier food choices and avoid eating when you are not hungry.

In cases of stress and anxiety and of depression, seeing a trained mental health professional can be helpful. In these cases, the mental health professional will often begin with behavioral therapy and will attempt to help you change your behaviors.

The mental health professional can then explore the emotions and thoughts underlying stress, anxiety, and depression and help you understand and control these emotions. Discussing your emotional issues and the problems you face every day with a mental health professional can be very helpful and can help you lose weight.

In some cases, the mental health professional will recommend psychiatric medication. Treatment of depressive symptoms with psychiatric medication can relieve depression, thereby stopping you from eating when you are not hungry, and can help you lose weight.[285]

Snacking

People who are overweight snack more often than people who are normal weight do.[286] Why then is snacking permitted in The Golden Gate Diet?

My clinical experiences with my patients have taught me that it is very difficult to get someone to stop snacking. It is, however, very possible to get someone to change what they are snacking on. Instead of snacking on high caloric density foods, you can snack on low caloric density foods. And while you can easily take in a lot of calories quickly by snacking on high caloric density foods such as chips and candy, if you snack on foods with a low caloric density, such as fruits and vegetables, you will not take in a lot of extra calories.

Snacking is by no means mandatory in The Golden Gate Diet. But feel free to snack in moderation. Just snack on healthy, low caloric density foods. Take a look at Alise's meal plans—they contain healthy snacks that taste so good.

Meal Timing

It may be worse to eat a big meal late in the day than to eat a big meal early in the day. Heavier people eat a greater fraction of their meals in the afternoon, evening, and night, while less heavy people eat earlier in the day.[287] Perhaps eating a somewhat large meal in the morning, by distending the stomach, causes you to feel full and not want to eat until much later—so while it may give you a lot of calories, it has the benefit of preventing you from eating shortly thereafter. In contrast, eating a large meal before you go to bed would not only give you a lot of calories, it would not prevent you from eating shortly thereafter, since you would not eat shortly thereafter anyway since you would be asleep, and it is not possible to prevent something that would not happen anyway.

So avoid eating large meals late in the day.

Sleep-Wake and Hunger-Satiety Rhythms

Overweight and obese people sleep less than normal weight people do.[288] On average, people who sleep 8 hours weigh the least, and for every hour less than 8 a person sleeps, her weight increases proportionately.[289]

Why is this?

There are several theories.

Experiments suggest that the sleep–wake cycle and the hunger–satiety cycle are intricately linked.

How does the body control hunger?

Part of the answer is a hormone called leptin. Leptin is produced mostly by fat cells, and fat cells secrete leptin into the blood.[290] Leptin then passes through the bloodstream until it reaches the brain, where it crosses the blood-brain barrier.[291]

A part of the brain called the hypothalamus controls both the appetite and wakefulness. When leptin reaches the hypothalamus, it stimulates the hypothalamic neurons (the brain cells of the hypothalamus). The stimulated hypothalamic neurons then decrease the feeling of hunger and appear to increase your metabolism.[292] This causes you to eat fewer calories and burn more calories and ultimately lose weight and lose fat.

So leptin may be an important "weight loss" hormone.

Another part of the answer is a hormone called ghrelin. Ghrelin is produced mostly by the stomach, and stomach cells secrete ghrelin into the blood.[293] Ghrelin then passes through the bloodstream until it reaches the brain, where it crosses the blood-brain barrier.[294] When ghrelin reaches the hypothalamus, it inhibits the hypothalamic neurons. The inhibited hypothalamic neurons then create the feeling of hunger and appear to decrease your metabolism. This causes you to eat more calories and burn fewer calories and ultimately gain weight and gain fat.[295]

So ghrelin may be an important "weight gain" hormone.

It turns out that the same hypothalamic neurons that control the appetite also may control feelings of sleepiness.[296] So by inhibiting these same hypothalamic neurons, ghrelin may not only control hunger, it may control sleep.[297] Ghrelin may both make you feel hungry and may make you sleep more.[298]

When you've been awake a long time, your body turns off production of leptin and turns on production of ghrelin.[299] It is possible that your body lowers your level of leptin and raises your level of ghrelin in order to make you feel sleepy and get you to go to sleep.

But if you don't listen to your body and go to sleep when you feel sleepy, with low levels of leptin and high levels of ghrelin you may not only feel tired, you may feel hungry. And you will eat and gain weight.*

Why is it that the cycles of satiety-hunger and sleepiness-wakefulness are intricately linked? Perhaps such interweaving of the two systems could help survival.

And it may be more profound than this: feelings of sexuality and other emotions may also be regulated by these hypothalamic pathways. So leptin and ghrelin may be pieces of the puzzle of how hunger, sleep, the sex drive, and other emotions are intertwined.

There is another, more prosaic theory for why people who sleep less weigh more. If you're up more, you have more hours to eat, since most people don't eat during sleep.

The bottom line: sleep eight hours a day—it may help you lose weight. If you're too busy to sleep eight hours a day, well, sleep when you can.

CASE STUDY Jonathan: Losing weight changed my life

When I was growing up, my family ate fattening foods. A typical dinner might be Southern fried chicken, French fries, and an ice cream sundae for dessert. I became overweight during childhood.

Later, I went to boarding school and had a difficult time fitting in with the other boys. They would make fun of me because I was so big.

As I entered adulthood, I would eat continually. I especially ate when I was unhappy or felt pressure at graduate school. Although I tried a number of diets, I continued to gain weight. This added further stress to my life because I felt guilty for harming my body.

Now, on the Golden Gate Diet, I have learned to eat 3 meals a day and 3 snacks rather than snacking all day long.

For me, a typical day on the Golden Gate Diet means a good-sized bowl of yogurt and fruit and a little bit of granola for breakfast. For a mid-morning snack, I might have carrots and hummus. For lunch, I might have salad and tuna fish. My second snack might be a piece of fruit—some grapes or an apple. For dinner I might have a salad, turkey, corn, vegetables, and nonfat pudding or pie for dessert.

Several things have helped me stick with the Golden Gate Diet. Before I started the Golden Gate Diet, on my way to school I used to pick up coffee and donuts for breakfast. I had thought the coffee and donuts would keep me awake and alert. Now, on the Golden Gate Diet, I eat breakfast at home and skip the donuts.

Sometimes I cook, and sometimes my girlfriend cooks. I encourage my girlfriend to cook healthy foods with a low caloric density.

Much to my surprise, I've lost 40 pounds. I feel better about myself. I've treated myself by going on a trip to Hawaii with my girlfriend.

Although I have had difficulties in relationships previously, I am now in a committed relationship. I feel more comfortable with myself, and I feel more comfortable with my performance in school.

---

* This is just a hypothesis! and certainly an oversimplification. Leptin and ghrelin are not diametrically opposed. Low levels of leptin might actually greatly increase rapid eye movement (REM) sleep while modestly decreasing slow wave sleep, and high levels of ghrelin may increase slow wave sleep. And doubtless many other factors interact with leptin and ghrelin in regulating sleep. Ghrelin may be important for short-term and long-term control of appetite, while the role of leptin might be confined to long-term control of appetite.

Chapter 14

Eating Disorders

Eating disorders are serious disturbances in eating behavior, such as a severe decrease in food intake.[300] People with eating disorders often have an excessive concern with body appearance or shape. Severe under-eating causes malnutrition, which can have serious physical consequences, including heart and kidney failure. People can die from heart and kidney failure as a result of malnutrition.

Eating disorders are more common in women than men: 85–95% of patients are women.

Eating disorders often coexist with other psychiatric illnesses, such as depression, anxiety disorders, substance abuse, and personality disorders.[301]

Anorexia Nervosa

Anorexia nervosa is a disease of severe under-eating. It is a common disease: it has been estimated that 0.3% of young women have anorexia nervosa.[302] Symptoms of anorexia include:[303]

- Refusal to maintain body weight at or above a minimally normal weight for age and height (<85% of normal)
- Failure to make expected weight gain during a period of growth (leading to body weight <85% of normal)
- Intense fear of gaining weight or becoming fat even though underweight
- Seeing oneself as fat when one is not fat, or undue influence of body weight or shape on self-evaluation
- Denial of the seriousness of the current very low body weight
- Failure to menstruate

People with anorexia often see themselves as being fat even though they are dangerously underweight.

The course of anorexia varies. Some people recover after a single episode, others alternate between periods of recovery and relapse of the disease, and others have a chronic course of decline. The annual death rate from anorexia is 0.6% per year.[304,305] The most common causes of death in people with anorexia are suicide and complications of alcoholism.[306,307]

Bulimia Nervosa

Bulimia nervosa is a disease of binge eating followed by behaviors to reduce weight. Like anorexia nervosa, it is a common disease: it has been estimated that 1% of young women and 0.1% of young men have bulimia nervosa.[308] Symptoms of bulimia include:[309]

- Recurrent episodes of binge eating
- Recurrent behavior to prevent weight gain, such as self-induced vomiting, misuse of laxatives or other medications, fasting, or excessive exercise
- Self-evaluation is unduly influenced by body shape and weight

People with bulimia are usually extremely unhappy with their physical appearance. They have intense shame about their purging activities and often conduct them in secrecy.

Binge Eating Disorder

Binge eating disorder is a disease of binge eating without the inappropriate behaviors to reduce weight of bulimia nervosa. It has been estimated that 1% of people have binge eating disorder.[310] Symptoms of binge eating disorder include:[311]

- Recurrent episodes of binge eating
- Marked distress regarding binge eating

Like people with bulimia, people with binge eating disorder are usually extremely unhappy with their physical appearance.[312] About 15% of people seeking weight loss treatment have binge eating disorder.[313]

Night Eating Syndrome

Night eating syndrome is an eating disorder in which patients lack appetite in the morning, eat excessively in the evening, feel tense and upset in the evening, and have insomnia.[314] Specifically patients who:

- Skip breakfast 4 or more times a week
- Eat more than half of their calories after 7 PM
- Have difficulty falling asleep more than 4 days a week

(These criteria are valid for American culture. Doctors in Mediterranean countries, where 25% of lean healthy people eat most of their food after 7 PM, define the syndrome as being present if patients eat more than half of their calories just before going to sleep or if they wake up in the middle of the night and eat half of their calories then.)[315]

Night eating syndrome affects about 1.5% of Americans.

Many people with night eating syndrome wake up in the middle of the night frequently. Often they feel under a compulsion to seek food. Many describe this as occurring when they are in a state of being half-asleep and half-awake. During this state most do not feel hungry but feel a need to swallow food.[316] Patients in this state feel that they are "out of control" and unable to stop eating.[317] Nearly half are sleep walkers. Depression and low self-esteem are common in people with night eating syndrome.[318]

Treatment of Eating Disorders

People with eating disorders need to be treated by a trained health professional. Treatment may include nutritional therapy, behavioral therapy, psychotherapy, and psychiatric medications. **This treatment often can make a big difference—psychiatric illness such as depression can be successfully treated, and anorectic and bulimic behaviors also can often be successfully treated.** Patients with night eating syndrome can be successfully treated with a drug called sertraline, which is a member of a class of drugs called selective serotonin reuptake inhibitors (SSRIs).[319]

Unfortunately, many people with anorexia or bulimia deny that they have an illness. Family members can be very helpful in convincing people with anorexia and bulimia to see a trained health professional and get appropriate care.

People who have had anorexia nervosa, bulimia nervosa, binge eating disorder, or night eating disorder should not attempt to lose weight on their own. If you have had or think you may now have any of these diseases, talk with your doctor, who can help you with a safe weight loss plan.

Chapter 15

Behavioral Therapy

Behavioral therapy can be a big help in losing weight. In behavioral therapy, people talk about their weight problem with a health professional—such as a psychiatrist, psychologist, social worker, nurse practitioner, or other trained mental health professional. The health professional gives the person suggestions about how to change their behaviors to lose weight. Behavioral therapy is a big help to obese people, but it can also help overweight people.

A special kind of behavioral therapy is called "cognitive behavioral therapy." Cognitive behavioral therapy attempts to change how people view eating. For example, it might change someone's views about the size of a healthy meal. Regularly meeting with a trained health professional can be very helpful in changing how people view food.

In cognitive behavioral therapy you discuss the positive reasons to lose weight (*e.g.*, it will improve my health ... it will make me look better) in order to reinforce these reasons in your mind. Cognitive behavioral therapy also reinforces your belief that you will succeed at weight loss.

One of the key concepts in cognitive behavioral therapy is **"people, places, things"**.

"People" means not eating with other people who are going to encourage you to eat. This might mean not eating with friends when you know they are going to go to McDonalds®.

"Places" means avoiding places where you will be tempted with high caloric density food, such as a Krispy Kreme® donut shop. "Places" also means going to places that serve healthier food, such as a vegetarian, Japanese, Italian, or Californian restaurant.

"Things" means avoiding things that stimulate the desire for high caloric density food. For example, the music from an ice cream truck will remind you of ice cream and can stimulate your desire for it.

Other helpful behavioral changes include avoiding situations where you snack too much. If you are watching television, don't have a bowl of potato chips with you! In general, you should try to keep food out of sight and out of reach. The Golden Gate Diet calls for 3 healthy meals a day and 3 healthy snacks a day to keep you full.

Coping skills can also be developed during behavioral therapy. For example, it can teach people how to cope successfully with difficult situations such as eating with other people who are eating a lot.

Sometimes people eat a lot when they get emotionally upset. Behavioral therapy can help people learn to avoid eating a lot when they are upset. It can also build up self-esteem, which can help someone stick to their diet.

Seeing a trained health professional—such as a psychiatrist, psychologist, social worker, nurse practitioner, or other trained health professional—can be a big help to obese people trying to lose weight. It can also be a big help to overweight people who have been trying unsuccessfully to lose weight.

Chapter 16

Drug Therapy for Obesity

If after 6 months of diet, exercise, and lifestyle changes you have not lost weight, you and your doctor should consider a trial of drug therapy. Drug therapy is only for:

- people with a BMI greater than 30
- people with a BMI greater than 27 who have either high blood pressure, diabetes, or high cholesterol.

The two drugs currently available for weight loss are Meridia® (sibutramine) and Xenical® (orlistat).

Meridia®

Meridia works directly on the appetite control center in the brain to suppress your appetite.[320] Meridia combined with a low calorie diet and exercise has been shown to help people lose weight and maintain weight loss. On average, people lose about 10 pounds after taking Meridia for a year.[321] Whether patients taking Meridia maintain their weight loss for longer periods of time is not known. The long-term side-effects of Meridia are also not known.

Many people cannot take Meridia. Meridia substantially increases the blood pressure in some patients, and blood pressure needs to be monitored carefully. Meridia can also cause a fast heart rate. Meridia should not be used by patients with a history of uncontrolled or poorly controlled high blood pressure, coronary artery disease, irregular heart rhythm, congestive heart failure, or stroke. Other patients who cannot take Meridia include patients who are taking monoamine oxidase inhibitors (which are a class of antidepressant medication), patients who have had anorexia nervosa or bulimia nervosa, and patients with severe liver or kidney disease. Patients who are planning to become pregnant, are pregnant, or are breast-feeding cannot use Meridia.

Meridia is a controlled substance. It can be abused and can cause physical or psychological dependence.

The most common side effects of Meridia are headache, dry mouth, loss of appetite, constipation, and insomnia.

People need to discuss their medical history with their doctors carefully before taking Meridia. Meridia helps some people lose weight, but it does not work for everyone.

For more information about Meridia, see the Meridia website (www.meridia.net).

Xenical®

Xenical acts in your digestive system to block about one third of the fat in your food from being digested. When taken with meals, it attaches to enzymes called lipases and prevents them from digesting fats. Undigested, the fats cannot be absorbed into the body and are passed out with the stool. Since one third of the fat you have eaten is not absorbed, Xenical will help you lose weight.[322] On average, after 2 years, people taking Xenical while following a diet lose 3–4% more weight than do people who are dieting without taking Xenical.[323] Whether patients taking Xenical maintain their weight loss for longer periods of time is not known. The long-term side effects of Xenical are also not known.

Xenical interferes with absorption of vitamins A, D, E, and K, so patients taking Xenical need to take a multi-vitamin at least 2 hours before or 2 hours after taking Xenical. Xenical should not be taken by patients who are pregnant, nursing, have food absorption problems, or have reduced bile flow.

Side effects of Xenical may include gas with an oily discharge, an increased number of bowel movements, an urgent need to have them, and an inability to control them. People need to discuss their medical histories with their doctors carefully before taking Xenical. Xenical helps some people lose weight, but it does not work for everyone.

For more information about Xenical, see the Xenical website (www.xenical.com).

Avoid Herbal Weight-Loss Medications

Herbal weight-loss medications have not been proven to promote weight loss in the long-term. In addition, they have serious side effects and are dangerous. The herbal medication Ephedra ("ma huang") has caused permanent disability and death in a number of people.[324] This includes cases of stroke and sudden cardiac death. Ephedra was recently banned by the FDA, although a federal judge overturned the ban. Sadly, the current law allows nutritional supplement companies to make false and sometimes dangerous claims about their products if they call them "foods" rather than "drugs". I can only hope that some of the members of congress reading my book will stand up to these nutritional supplement companies, who are the snake oil salesmen of the modern era.

Why the CDC, FDA, and FTC can't protect you from nutritional supplements

Make no mistake. The Centers for Disease Control and Prevention, the Food and Drug Administration, and the Federal Trade Commission are the good guys. They want to protect the public.

Why can't they stop the lies? Why can't they ban the bogus diet products?

You can thank the 4 billion dollar nutritional supplement industry. In 1994, under intense pressure from the nutritional supplement industry, Congress tied the hands of the FDA: the FDA is not allowed to ban nutritional supplements until a particular supplement directly harms many people. Nutritional supplements that are harmless but that do not do what they claim to do cannot be banned. That means that companies selling bogus diet pills can advertise their products and can claim their products cause weight loss, even if it's untrue.

Do the lobbyists for the nutritional supplement companies spend millions of dollars to emasculate the FDA? You bet they do.[325]

Chapter 17

WEIGHT-REDUCTION SURGERY

Weight-reduction surgery (bariatric surgery) causes dramatic weight loss. There are risks to the surgery, and you can have problems after the surgery. It is healthier and safer to lose weight by diet and exercise than by weight-reduction surgery. Most people should make a serious attempt at weight loss by diet and exercise for 6 months before considering weight-reduction surgery. With the diet described in this book you can succeed and avoid a potentially dangerous surgery that has long-term problems associated with it. That said, if after 6 months you are still severely obese, you should consider weight-reduction surgery.

Weight-reduction surgery is effective and produces sustained weight loss in most patients. Gastric bypass is the most commonly performed weight-reduction operation in the United States. People with a BMI over 40 lose on average 40 to 70 pounds after gastric bypass.[326] It is clear that much of the weight stays off. However, some studies found that over the course of 10 years, half of the weight is gained back, while other studies found that almost none of the weight is gained back.[327] The good news is that diseases caused by too much fat, such as diabetes, become less severe after weight loss surgery.

While it is clear that people with a BMI greater than 40 lose more weight after gastric bypass surgery than from medical treatment, the data is less clear-cut for people with a BMI between 35 and 40.[328] The data for people with a BMI between 35 and 40 points to surgery being superior to medical therapy but is not conclusive.

The risk of death from the gastric bypass operation is about 1%.[329] Over time, untreated severe obesity has a much higher death rate.

After surgery, patients have less depression and improved self-esteem.[330] Usually marital satisfaction increases after surgery; however, divorce is not uncommon.[331]

Weight-reduction surgery is only for:

- people with extreme obesity (BMI greater than 40)
- people with severe obesity (BMI greater than 35) and serious obesity-related illness (for example, diabetes)

Patients with a psychiatric disturbance should undergo psychiatric evaluation prior to surgery, since patients with a severe psychiatric disorder may not have a good outcome from the surgery.

By far the most common weight-reduction operation performed in the United States is the gastric bypass with Roux-en-Y reconstruction. In this operation the stomach is stapled so that the new stomach pouch is only 50 milliliters (about the size of 2 ounces of water). In addition, part of the small intestine, which normally absorbs food and nutrients, is bypassed. With a smaller stomach pouch, most people stop becoming hungry after eating a relatively small amount of food.[332] With part of the small intestine bypassed, less food and nutrients are absorbed into the body.

The gastric bypass operation results in greater weight loss than another weight-reduction operation, vertical banded gastroplasty. I recommend that patients wanting weight reduction surgery go to a surgeon who does the gastric bypass operation and do not go to a surgeon who does only vertical banded gastroplasty.

The gastric bypass operation can be done "open", with an incision from the lower part of the ribcage to the bellybutton, or it can be done "laparoscopically", with multiple small incisions. There is no significant difference in the death rate after surgery between the open and laparoscopic procedures.[333] The problems after the open and laparoscopic approaches differ somewhat, but neither approach appears to be dramatically better than the other.[334] However, people return to their normal activities faster with the laparoscopic approach.[335]

It is important to remember that this is major surgery. This is true even if the operation is done laparoscopically with multiple small incisions—just because the incisions are small does not mean the operation is small. Patients who are extremely obese are more likely to experience serious problems after major surgery. In addition to the death rate of about 1%, 20% of patients experience complications (that is, significant problems). These complications include wound infections, disruption of the abdominal wall, leaks from where the bowel was reconnected, blood clots in the leg veins ("deep vein thrombosis"), and lung problems. The most serious complications are staple line leak and deep vein thrombosis. Patients with a staple line leak need to be taken back to surgery on an emergency basis to fix the leak.

Patients who are dramatically obese (BMI>50) have a greater chance of serious problems and of dying from the surgery than patients who are less obese (BMI 40–50).[336] Of course, patients who are dramatically obese, in general, are the patients who need the surgery the most.

After weight-reduction surgery you will have to be monitored for complications of the surgery for the rest of your life. After the surgery, patients do not absorb iron, vitamin B_{12}, calcium, vitamin D, and vitamin A well. Patients need life-long supplementation of these minerals and vitamins to avoid anemia (iron and vitamin B$_{12}$), osteoporosis (calcium and vitamin D), and blindness (vitamin A).[337] Up to 10% of patients develop wound hernias, and 2% develop bowel obstruction due to the formation of scar tissue within the abdomen. Other long-term complications that can occur are excess weight loss with malnutrition and failure to lose enough weight. Also, some patients experience a "dumping syndrome," with symptoms of rapid heart beat and nausea after eating foods with a high sugar content.

For more information about weight loss surgery, talk with your doctor or visit the website of the American Society for Bariatric Surgery (www.asbs.org).

Chapter 18

Conclusion: why People Succeed on the Golden Gate Diet

Before you started the Golden Gate Diet, it was easy to thumb through the pages of *Cosmo* and look at a thin, beautiful model and fall into a state of defeatism. You may have had these thoughts: "I can never look that way. I was just not born with that body."

But as you now know, the truth is quite different. What distinguishes the girl in *Cosmo* from people who are heavier is that that girl is eating fewer calories and burning more calories.

She's eating fewer calories in one of two ways. She's either starving herself—needlessly—or she's eating foods with a low caloric density, whether she knows it or not.

And she's burning more calories by going to the gym every day.

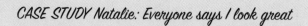

CASE STUDY Natalie: Everyone says I look great

When I was a teenager, I was thin. Then I started college and I put on the "freshman fifteen". Oh boy. I continued to gain weight during college. For the last five years I have been working at an internet firm in San Francisco, and you get really busy. I work hard and play hard. It makes it hard to diet.

I got up to 160 pounds.

Then Dr. Brook introduced me to the Golden Gate Diet. It's so easy to follow. I like the food. Cereal. Fruit. Bananas. Scrambled egg whites with cream cheese. Yogurt. A thick smoothie. Pizza with nonfat mozzarella. Turkey burgers. Curried chicken salad. Spinach salad. A roast beef sandwich. Spaghetti with marinara sauce. Japanese noodles. Fresh fish. Grilled tuna. Salmon. Barbequed chicken. Sometimes sirloin steak! Corn. Grilled tomatoes. String beans. Squash. Mashed potatoes. Blueberry pie. Chocolate pudding. Angel food cake. A glass of wine almost every day. The best thing about it is it's all healthy food. I've been exercising, and I've really gotten into shape. I am very strong now. I look good, and I feel good.

I weigh 120 pounds. It's amazing how people treat you differently when you lose weight. And I don't just mean men—that's obvious. When I go into a store to buy something, the saleswoman treats me differently.

Everybody says I'm cute. I love the attention. It's so much fun.

People succeed at the Golden Gate Diet because they are doing similar things. And no, I don't mean they are starving themselves! They eat food with low caloric density and stay away from the fattening food with high caloric density. There is no magic here. They enjoy the food they eat. They eat fruits and vegetables instead of potato chips and Cheetos®, they eat fish and skinless chicken instead of prime rib and *foie gras*, they eat pie instead of cake. They drink red wine instead of hard liquor, and they don't overdo it! And they go to the gym.

So there's no magic here.

The Golden Gate Diet makes it easy. The meal plans are delicious and have helped countless people lose weight. And the tables in the book listing the caloric density of almost every food in the American diet make it easy to know what foods are safe to eat, and what foods are not.

You can have the body that you want by following the Golden Gate Diet. As you lose weight, you will feel good about yourself.

You will love the compliments everyone gives you about having lost weight.

You know how to lose weight, and you know you can always keep your weight down.

And you won't just look great. By eating healthy you'll add years to your life. Because the Golden Gate Diet lowers your risk for heart disease and your risk for cancer.

What is the Golden Gate Diet really? It is the scientific way to lose weight and eat healthy. From clinical experience and studies of thousands of patients, we have learned what foods cause someone to gain weight and what foods cause someone to lose weight, what foods cause heart disease and what foods prevent heart disease, what foods cause cancer and what foods prevent cancer. This experience and knowledge allowed me to design a rational way to lose weight, and I have shown that it works for my patients.

The Golden Gate Diet is the way to eat healthy.

There's no magic here, only science.

Part Two

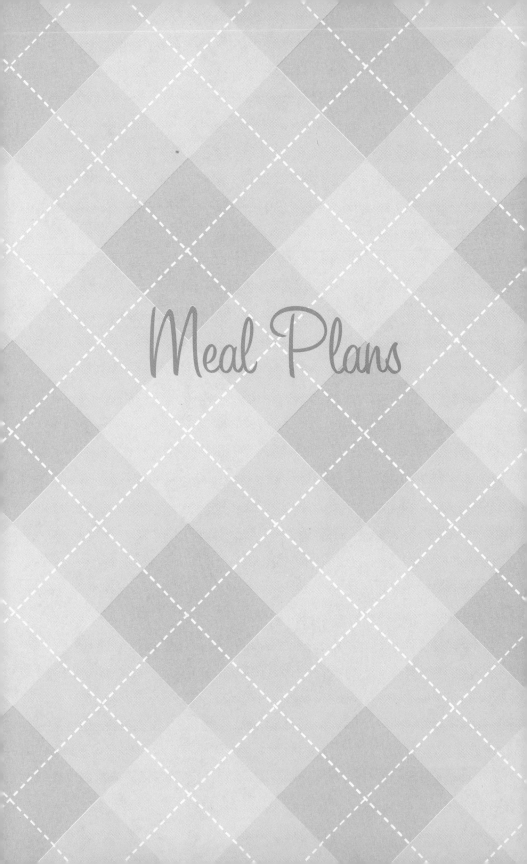

Meal Plans

It is important to remember that there are 2 stages to the diet. During the first stage you lose weight at a rate of 1–2 pounds a week until you reach your goal weight. During the second stage—the maintenance stage—you neither gain nor lose weight, but maintain a stable weight.

Included below are 2 different three week meal plans. The first plan is a 1200 calories a day plan (for weight loss), and the second plan is a 2000 calories a day plan (for weight maintenance). Feel free to modify these plans. They are meant to give you an idea of the sorts of foods you can eat, but you can eat different foods—just make sure they have a low caloric density!

For example, suppose you are on the Thursday afternoon of week 2 of the 1200 calories a day plan (for weight loss). The recommended afternoon snack is nonfat yogurt with fruit, which contains 213 calories. But you don't like yogurt, you like cottage cheese. Then by all means substitute a cup of nonfat cottage cheese (123 calories) and ½ a cup of blueberries (41 calories) for the yogurt.

Just make sure to substitute items that have a similar number of calories. What's important is that the total number of calories for the day is about the same, that the foods all have a low caloric density, and that you space the calories out through the course of the day. (Don't have 1000 calories for breakfast and 200 calories for the rest of the day—you'll get hungry.)

Feel free to look through the tables in this book to help you make substitutions—the tables show the caloric density and number of calories of practically every food known to man.

Please note that the number of calories listed for each food is from the USDA.[338,339,340]

The 1200 Calories a Day Plan (for Weight Loss)

Start off by following the meal plans—each is about 1200 calories a day.
If you are losing 1–2 pounds a week, 1200 calories is just right—stick with the 1200 calories meal plan.

If you are losing less than 1 pound a week, you need to eat less than 1200 calories. The easiest way to do this is to decrease your portion size *gradually*.

If you are losing more than 2 pounds a week, you are losing weight too quickly. The easiest way to do this is to increase your portion size *gradually*.

Sunday, week 1, breakfast

Herbed scrambled egg substitute (½ cup, 53 calories) or egg white—scramble in
1 tablespoon nonfat cream cheese (15 calories) and chopped mixed herbs
A banana (109 calories)
A cup of coffee with skim milk and NutraSweet

Snack

White bean spread
6 baby carrots (24 calories)
Water

Lunch

Turkey burger made with nonfat turkey (193 calories)
Place on mixed greens and top with tomato, sautéed onion, Dijon mustard, and
nonfat mayo
A sweet pickle (16 calories)
Diet soda (4 calories)

Make sure you get some exercise today.

Snack

Unsweetened apple sauce (½ cup, 53 calories)

Dinner

Butternut squash soup with 1 tablespoon sour cream and chopped chives (1 cup,
140 calories)
Braised veal chop with mushrooms and peppers (259 calories)
8 asparagus spears roasted with balsamic vinegar (28 calories)
Water with lemon

Snack

An orange (69 calories)

Monday, week 1, breakfast

Raisin bran cereal with skim milk (1 cup cereal with ½ cup milk, 229 calories)
Tomato juice (41 calories)
If desired, a cup of coffee with skim milk and flavored with NutraSweet

If you can, go running today.

Snack

Blueberries (½ cup, 41 calories)

Lunch

Turkey sandwich—add arugula, roasted red peppers, and low fat pesto mayo (420 calories)
Apple coleslaw (½ cup, 42 calories)
Diet soda (4 calories)

Snack

Smoothie—1 banana, ½ cup nonfat yogurt, and 2 strawberries

Dinner

Seared halibut kabobs with lemon (238 calories)
Italian vegetable stew (150 calories)
½ cup brown rice (108 calories)
Water with cucumber slices

Snack

Low calorie jello

Tuesday, week 1, breakfast

Low fat French toast (2 slices, 252 calories) with blueberries (½ cup, 41 calories)
2 vegetarian breakfast links (63 calories)
If desired a cup of coffee with skim milk and flavored with NutraSweet

If you can, go to the gym today.

Snack

Half an apple sliced (41 calories) drizzled with 2 tablespoons nonfat vanilla yogurt

Lunch

A can of light tuna, with mixed in low fat mayonnaise, chopped scallion, dill, celery, and lemon juice, stuffed into 2 tomato halves (410 calories)
Water or diet soda

Snack

Waldorf fruit salad with fresh apples, mixed fruit, nonfat mayonnaise, ground nutmeg, raisins, and chopped walnuts (⅓ cup, 70 calories)

Dinner

Minestrone soup (82 calories)
Zucchini pasta "lasagne" with nonfat mozzarella (230 calories)
Green beans with balsamic vinegar (110 calories)
Water with lemon

Snack

nonfat chocolate pudding (½ cup, 107 calories)

Wednesday, week 1, breakfast

Muesli cereal "parfait"—Muesli (⅔ cup, 190 calories) layered with yogurt and 4 sliced strawberries (16 calories)
If desired a cup of coffee with skim milk and flavored with NutraSweet

Try to go running today.

Snack

Honeydew melon (⅛ melon, 56 calories) with nonfat cottage cheese (¼ cup, 31 calories)

Lunch

Curried chicken salad with grapes in lettuce wrap (280 calories)
Water or diet soda

Snack

Eggplant dip (½ cup, 40 calories) with celery sticks (1 stalk, 6 calories)

Dinner

Chopped vegetable salad (100 calories)
Fettuccine with roasted vegetables (225 calories)
Water

Snack

Strawberry granita (120 calories)

Thursday, week 1, breakfast

2 low fat waffles (166 calories)
A glass of skim milk (86 calories)
If desired, a cup of coffee with skim milk and flavored with NutraSweet

Try to go to the gym today.

Snack

Roasted artichoke with Dijon dipping sauce (nonfat mayo, Dijon mustard, and lemon juice) (57 calories)

Lunch

Nicoise salad—3 ounces canned light tuna in water atop mixed greens, green beans, 1 sliced baby potato, red onion, black olives, 2 cherry tomatoes, and light vinaigrette (293 calories)
Water or diet soda

Snack

Citrus baked apple with nonfat vanilla yogurt (140 calories)

Dinner

Gazpacho (28 calories)
Poached salmon (6 ounces, 368 calories) with nonfat cucumber dill yogurt sauce
Sautéed carrot and zucchini strips

Snack

Rice pudding (½ cup, 184 calories)

Friday, week 1, breakfast

Oatmeal (1 cup, 145 calories) with cinnamon and 1 teaspoon drizzle maple syrup
½ cup mixed berries (30 calories)
If desired a cup of coffee with skim milk and flavored with NutraSweet

Try to go running today.

Snack

4 tablespoons of hummus (92 calories) and 8 baby carrots (32 calories)

Lunch

Sliced turkey lettuce wrap with 1 sliced avocado, tomato, and nonfat mayonnaise (140 calories)
Diet soda (4 calories)

Snack

An orange (62 calories)

Dinner

Chicken and vegetable stir-fry (290 calories)
½ cup brown rice (108 calories)
Water

Snack

Pumpkin pie (1 piece, 229 calories)

Saturday, week 1, breakfast

2 pancakes prepared from lower calorie mix (148 calories): add ½ cup blueberries to mix (41 calories)
If desired a cup of coffee with skim milk and flavored with NutraSweet

Snack

Banana smoothie: blend 1 cup orange juice, 1 cup vanilla low fat yogurt, and a banana (206 calories)

Lunch

Roast beef sandwich (346 calories) with grilled red onion, Dijon mustard, and horseradish sauce
A sweet pickle (18 calories)
Sugar-free lemonade (5 calories)

Don't forget to exercise today.

Snack

A peach (42 calories)

Dinner

Orange and cumin glazed salmon with ½ cup toasted couscous (431 calories)
Sesame broccoli and carrots (73 calories)
Water with lemon

Snack

Red wine poached pear (150 calories)

Sunday, week 2, breakfast

3 low fat waffles (4" waffles, 249 calories)
6 strawberries (24 calories)
If desired a cup of coffee with skim milk and flavored with NutraSweet

Snack

Cantaloupe with nonfat cottage cheese (1/8 melon, 24 calories and ½ cup cottage cheese, 62 calories)

Lunch

Warm bay scallop salad with tomatoes and chopped basil on baby spinach (110 calories)
Water with lemon

Snack

10 frozen grapes (36 calories)

Dinner

Eye of round roast, fat cut away (6 ounces, 286 calories) with roasted red pepper sauce (25 calories)
Roasted ratatouille (91 calories)

Snack

Blueberry pie (1 piece, 271 calories)

Monday, week 2, breakfast

Raisin bran cereal (1 cup, 186 calories) with skim milk (½ cup, 43 calories)
A glass of skim milk (86 calories)
If desired a cup of coffee with skim milk and flavored with NutraSweet

Try to go running today.

Snack

Cucumber slices topped with baby shrimp (6 ounces, 204 calories)

Lunch

Waldorf chicken salad on mixed greens with apples, walnuts, and nonfat
mayonnaise (310 calories)
Lemonade sweetened with NutraSweet (5 calories)

Snack

A pear (98 calories)

Dinner

Minestrone soup (1 cup, 82 calories)
Potato gnocchi with marinara sauce (1 cup, 340 calories)
Squash (¾ cup, 60 calories)
Water

Snack

Sugar-free jello (½ cup, 8 calories)

Tuesday, week 2, breakfast

Egg substitute (1 cup, 106 calories) omelette with 2 slices of nonfat cheese (62 calories) and mushrooms
A glass of tomato juice (41 calories)
If desired a cup of coffee with skim milk and flavored with NutraSweet

Go to the gym today.

Snack

A tangerine (37 calories)

Lunch

Thai rice noodle salad with shrimp, bean sprouts, cucumber, mint, lime, and chili sauce (241 calories)
Diet soda (4 calories)

Snack

An apple (68 calories)

Dinner

Barbequed skinless chicken breast (320 calories)
Vegetarian baked beans (¾ cup, 177 calories)
Apple and carrot coleslaw
Sauteéd spinach (1 cup, 53 calories)
Water

Snack

Grilled fruit kabob with honeyed yogurt

Wednesday, week 2, breakfast

Muesli cereal parfait (⅔ cup, 190 calories) with yogurt (½ cup, 44 calories) and sliced strawberries
If desired a cup of coffee with skim milk and flavored with NutraSweet

Go running today.

Snack

Half a mango (68 calories)

Lunch

Turkey chili with 2 slices avocado (243 calories)
Water or diet soda

Snack

A frozen banana (109 calories)
Dinner
Vegetable soup (1 cup, 72 calories)
Grilled skinless turkey breast (6 ounces, 266 calories) with cranberry-orange compote (112 calories)
Roasted broccoli (¾ cup, 19 calories)
Water

Snack

Nonfat tapioca pudding (½ cup, 98 calories)

Thursday, week 2, breakfast

Cream of wheat (1 cup, 133 calories)
Raspberries (¾ cup, 45 calories)
A glass of skim milk (86 calories)
If desired, a cup of coffee with skim milk and flavored with NutraSweet

Go to the gym today.

Snack

A banana (109 calories)

Lunch

Grilled Portobello sandwich with roasted red pepper, baby spinach, and low fat pesto mayo (260 calories)

Snack

Nonfat yogurt with fruit (8 ounces, 213 calories)

Dinner

Broiled herb-crusted trout with lemon (6 ounces, 206 calories)
A sweet potato (164 calories)
Brussels sprouts (1 cup, 65 calories)
A glass of wine if desired (3.5 ounces, 74 calories)
Water

Snack

Boston cream pie (1 piece, 232 calories)

Friday, week 2, breakfast

Egg whites scrambled with salsa and 2 slices avocado (260 calories)
A glass of skim milk (86 calories)
If desired a cup of coffee with skim milk and flavored with NutraSweet

Go running today.

Snack

Sliced apple (81 calories) with spiced nonfat yogurt dip

Lunch

Turkey and black bean chili on couscous with shredded nonfat cheddar (259 calories)
Iced tea sweetened with NutraSweet (7 calories)
Water

Snack

2 apricots (34 calories)

Dinner

Carrot ginger soup (120 calories)
Broiled chicken breast (284 calories) with roasted tomato salsa (22 calories)
Mashed potatoes (⅓ cup, 83 calories)
Butternut squash purée (1 cup, 94 calories)

Snack

Nonfat vanilla pudding (½ cup, 105 calories)

Saturday, week 2, breakfast

2 pancakes prepared from low calorie mix (148 calories)
Half a grapefruit (39 calories)
A glass of skim milk (86 calories)
If desired a cup of coffee with skim milk and flavored with NutraSweet

Don't forget to exercise today.

Snack

White bean dip with 6 green beans

Lunch

Spaghetti with chunky tomato sauce and cubed chicken breast (290 calories)
Lemonade sweetened with NutraSweet

Snack

An apple (81 calories)

Dinner

Grilled shrimp skewer with pineapple and bell peppers (350 calories)
Rice (½ cup, 103 calories)
Grilled green beans
A glass of wine if desired (3.5 ounces, 74 calories)
Water

Snack

Watermelon (one wedge, 92 calories)

Sunday, week 3, breakfast

Egg white scramble with dill and 1 tablespoon nonfat sour cream (270 calories)
A glass of skim milk (86 calories)
If desired a cup of coffee with skim milk and flavored with NutraSweet

Snack

Honeydew melon or cantaloupe (⅛ melon, 56 calories)

Lunch

Moroccan sliced chicken breast salad with olives, figs, and sliced orange on mixed greens (290 calories)
Low calorie lemonade
Water

Snack

A peach (42 calories)

Dinner

Black bean soup (100 calories)
Vegetable and turkey soft tacos with salsa and nonfat sour cream (300 calories)
Diet soda or water

Snack

Nonfat pudding

Monday, week 3, breakfast

High fiber cereal with skim milk and blueberries (1 cup cereal and ½ cup milk, 269 calories total)

If desired a cup of coffee with skim milk and flavored with NutraSweet

Go running today.

Snack

Nonfat yogurt with fruit (8 ounces, 213 calories)

Lunch

Spinach salad with roasted pear, toasted pecans, and sliced grilled turkey breast (390 calories)

Diet soda, tea, or coffee

Water with lemon

Snack

A sliced apple (81 calories) drizzled with 2 tablespoons nonfat vanilla yogurt

Dinner

Grilled chicken skewers marinated in yogurt, cumin, lemon, and mint (260 calories)

Sweet white corn (1 ear, 83 calories)

Carrot and orange salad

Water with cucumber

Snack

Pineapple grilled with lemon and honey (70 calories)

Tuesday, week 3, breakfast

2 slices of French toast made with egg substitute, nonfat milk, cinnamon, and vanilla (252 calories)
2 figs (97 calories)
If desired a cup of coffee with skim milk and flavored with NutraSweet

Go to the gym today.

Snack

4 tablespoons of hummus (92 calories) and 8 baby carrots (32 calories)

Lunch

Salmon burger with baby spinach, tomato, and Dijon on half a whole wheat pita (220 calories)
Cucumber salad (36 calories)
Diet soda, tea, or coffee (5 calories)
Water

Snack

10 grapes (36 calories)

Dinner

Bell peppers stuffed with low fat ground turkey (180 calories)
Mashed potatoes
Steamed baby carrots
Water

Snack

Sugar-free jello (5 calories)

Wednesday, week 3, breakfast

Cream of wheat cereal (1 cup, 133 calories) with orange slices and cinnamon
A glass of skim milk (86 calories)
Coffee with skim milk

Go running today.

Snack

A banana (109 calories)

Lunch

Mixed greens salad with grilled shrimp, black beans, roasted corn, and red bell pepper (320 calories)
Diet soda, tea, or coffee
Water

Snack

Nonfat yogurt with NutraSweet (98 calories)

Dinner

Mixed greens salad
Baked eggplant and zucchini parmesan (without breading) with tomato sauce and nonfat mozzarella (260 calories)
Diet soda or water

Snack

Grilled pineapple (¾ cup, 58 calories)

Thursday, week 3, breakfast

Corn and zucchini omelette with egg substitute (¾ cup, 159 calories) or egg whites with salsa
A glass of skim milk (86 calories)
8 strawberries (32 calories)
If desired a cup of coffee with skim milk and flavored with NutraSweet

Go to the gym today.

Snack

Hummus (¼ cup, 92 calories)
Cucumber slices (10 calories)

Lunch

Japanese soba noodle salad with snow peas, carrots, peas, mushrooms, and scallion (310 calories)
Iced green tea
Water

Snack

Roasted corn on the cob

Dinner

Linguini with white clam sauce (1 ½ cups, 245 calories)
Sautéed spinach (1 cup, 53 calories)
Water
A plum (36 calories)

Snack

Nonfat chocolate pudding (4 ounces, 107 calories) with 6 raspberries

Friday, week 3, breakfast

Oatmeal (1 cup, 145 calories) with cinnamon and blueberries (½ cup, 41 calories)

A glass of tomato juice (41 calories)

If desired a cup of coffee with skim milk and flavored with NutraSweet

Go running today.

Snack

2 plums (72 calories)

Lunch

Chinese chicken salad—chopped grilled chicken breast, tangerine, sliced almonds, bean sprouts, and orange vinaigrette (210 calories)

Diet soda, coffee, or tea

Water

Iced green tea

Snack

6 strawberries (24 calories)

Dinner

Jicama-apple salad with bell pepper and lemon

Herb crusted grilled trout with lime (6 ounces, 288 calories)

Grilled shiitake mushrooms (1 cup, 80 calories)

A baked potato (145 calories) with salsa

Water

Snack

Nonfat chocolate pudding with ½ sliced banana

Saturday, week 3, breakfast

Scrambled egg substitute (¾ cup, 159 calories) with chopped spinach, mushrooms, and tomato
A glass of skim milk (86 calories)
If desired, a cup of coffee with skim milk and flavored with NutraSweet

Snack

A banana (109 calories)

Lunch

Sweet and sour chicken with vegetables (350 calories)
½ cup brown rice (108 calories)
Iced tea sweetened with NutraSweet
Water

Snack

10 grapes (36 calories)

Dinner

Tomato basil salad
Grilled sirloin steak fat cut away (6 ounces, 332 calories) with horseradish sauce (nonfat sour cream, horseradish, and Dijon mustard)
Mashed potatoes (⅓ cup, 66 calories)
8 asparagus spears (28 calories)
Water

Snack

Citrus baked apple

The 2000 Calories a Day Plan (for Weight Maintenance)

Use the 2000 calories a day plan to maintain a stable weight. Again, everyone is different—some people are bigger, some people are smaller, some people exercise frequently, some people are not very active. For some people 2000 calories will cause them to gain weight—for many people 2000 will be the right number of calories and will not cause them to gain or lose weight—and for some people 2000 calories will cause them to lose weight.

How do you tell if 2000 is too much, too little, or just right? Weigh yourself!

If you are at your goal weight and you are neither gaining nor losing weight on the 2000 calories a day plan, then 2000 calories is just right—stick with the 2000 calories meal plan.

If you are at your goal weight, and you are losing weight on the 2000 calories a day plan, then 2000 calories is not enough. You need to increase the number of calories you are consuming. You can either increase your portion size *gradually* or add a few more foods *gradually*.

If you are at your goal weight but you are gaining weight on the 2000 calories a day plan, then 2000 calories a day is too much. Decrease your portion size *gradually*.

Sunday, week 1, breakfast

Scrambled egg substitute (½ cup) or egg white: scramble in 2 pieces of nonfat American cheese (168 calories)—top with salsa and 2 slices of avocado
Orange banana smoothie: blend 1 banana, an 8 ounce glass of orange juice, and 1 cup vanilla low fat yogurt (206 calories)
If desired, a cup of coffee with skim milk and flavored with NutraSweet

Make sure you get some exercise today.

Snack

Hummus (6 tablespoons, 138 calories), tahini (1 tablespoon, 89 calories), 5 black olives (25 calories), and ½ piece of whole wheat pita (83 calories)
Water with lemon

Lunch

Turkey burger made with nonfat turkey (193 calories), place on mixed greens and top with tomato, sautéed mushrooms, onions, and Dijon mustard
A sweet pickle (16 calories)
Diet soda (4 calories)

Snack

12 macadamia nuts (203 calories)

Dinner

Butternut squash soup (1 cup, 78 calories)
Braised veal cutlet with mushrooms and peppers (6 ounces, 358 calories)
Mashed potatoes, preferably made with water or skim milk, no butter or margarine! (¾ cup, 122 calories)
Spinach sauté
A glass of red wine (3.5 ounces, 74 calories)
Water

Snack

Nonfat vanilla pudding (½ cup, 105 calories)

Monday, week 1, breakfast

Raisin bran cereal with skim milk (1 cup cereal with ½ cup milk, 229 calories)
Blueberries (½ cup, 41 calories)
If desired a cup of coffee with skim milk and flavored with NutraSweet

If you can, go running today.

Snack

Waldorf fruit salad with fresh apples, mixed fruit, low fat mayonnaise, ground nutmeg, raisins, and chopped walnuts (⅓ cup, 70 calories)

Lunch

Turkey wrap: add lettuce, tomatoes, roasted red pepper, onions, low fat mayonnaise, preferably lower calorie whole wheat tortilla bread (320 calories)
Apple coleslaw
An orange (62 calories)
Diet soda (4 calories)

Snack

Grilled artichoke with dipping sauce (nonfat mayonnaise, Dijon mustard, and lemon juice) (1 medium artichoke, 60 calories)
Water

Dinner

Grilled tuna kebab with mango salsa (236 calories)
Rice (½ cup, 103 calories)
Zucchini "pasta" with 1 tablespoon olive oil (70 calories)
A glass of white wine if desired (3.5 ounces, 70 calories)
Water

Snack

Apple cinnamon crumble (356 calories)

Tuesday, week 1, breakfast

Low fat French toast (2 slices, 252 calories)
Reduced calorie pancake syrup (2 tablespoons, 50 calories)
Blueberries (½ cup, 41 calories)
2 vegetarian breakfast links (63 calories)
A glass of orange juice (8 ounces, 112 calories)
If desired a cup of coffee with skim milk and flavored with NutraSweet

If you can, go to the gym today.

Snack

Half an apple, sliced (41 calories)
Natural peanut butter (2 tablespoons, 188 calories)

Lunch

A can of light tuna with mixed in nonfat mayonnaise, chopped scallion, dill,
celery, and lemon juice stuffed into 2 tomato halves
Water or diet soda

Snack

Unsweetened apple sauce (½ cup, 53 calories)

Dinner

Vegetable soup (130 calories)
Skinless grilled chicken breast with barbecue sauce (308 calories) and ½ grilled
peach (½ cup, 179 calories)
Yellow corn (1 ear, 83 calories)
Potato salad (½ cup, 179 calories)
Carrot jicama salad
A glass of red wine (74 calories)
Water

Snack

Mixed berries (1 cup, 60 calories) with nonfat sour cream (2 tablespoons, 24
calories)

Wednesday, week 1, breakfast

Muesli cereal "parfait" (2/3 cup, 190 calories) with nonfat vanilla yogurt (½ cup, 44 calories) and sliced banana
If desired a cup of coffee with skim milk and flavored with NutraSweet

Try to go running today.

Snack

Honeydew melon with nonfat cottage cheese (⅛ melon, 56 calories, and ½ cup cottage cheese, 62 calories)

Lunch

Curried chicken salad with grapes, scallion, nonfat mayonnaise in lettuce wrap (260 calories)
Water or diet soda

Snack

Nonfat chocolate pudding (4 ounces, 107 calories) with sliced toasted almonds

Dinner

Vegetable antipasto (66 calories)
Spaghetti with chunky tomato basil sauce and roasted veggies (270 calories)
Mashed butternut squash (1 cup, 94 calories)
A glass of chianti, if desired (74 calories)
Water

Snack

A piece of angel food cake (72 calories)

Thursday, week 1, breakfast

1 slice of toast with 1 tablespoon natural peanut butter, 1 tablespoon low calorie jam (116 calories), and ½ sliced banana
A glass of orange juice (112 calories)
A glass of skim milk (86 calories)
If desired a cup of coffee with skim milk and flavored with NutraSweet

Try to go to the gym today.

Snack

Vanilla nonfat yogurt with ½ chopped apple and raisins (140 calories)

Lunch

Turkey/black bean chili with 1 tablespoon shredded nonfat cheese (270 calories)
An apple (81 calories)
Water or diet soda

Snack

Nonfat chocolate pudding (107 calories) with 1 tablespoon sliced almonds

Dinner

Lentil soup (80 calories)
Baby spinach topped with grilled salmon, cucumber, tomato, and dill dressing (247 calories)
A glass of red wine (3½ ounces, 70 calories)

Snack

A piece of cherry pie (304 calories)

Friday, week 1, breakfast

Oatmeal (1 cup, 145 calories) with a sliced banana (109 calories) and cinnamon

Apricot-pineapple smoothie (225 calories)

2 vegetarian breakfast links (63 calories)

If desired a cup of coffee with skim milk and flavored with NutraSweet

Try to go running today.

Snack

4 tablespoons of hummus (92 calories) with asparagus spears (28 calories) and 8 baby carrots (32 calories)

Lunch

Sliced turkey sandwich with tomatoes, cranberry sauce, and nonfat mayonnaise (320 calories)

Diet soda (4 calories)

Snack

Roasted corn on the cob (90 cal)

Dinner

Tomato basil soup (120 calories)

Braised skinless (grilled) chicken breast (284 calories) with artichoke hearts (120 calories) and tomato (26 calories)

8 asparagus spears (28 calories)

A glass (3½ ounces) of red wine (74 calories)

Water

Snack

Light yellow cake (one piece, 181 calories)

Saturday, week 1, breakfast

2 pancakes prepared from lower calorie mix (148 calories) with a mashed banana (109 calories) and cinnamon added to the mixture
Low calorie syrup (2 tablespoons, 50 calories)
If desired, a cup of coffee with skim milk and flavored with NutraSweet

Snack

12 macadamia nuts (203 calories)

Lunch

Roast beef sandwich (346 calories) with horseradish, Dijon sauce and grilled onions
A sweet pickle (16 calories)
Potato salad (½ cup, 179 calories)
Sugar-free lemonade (5 calories)

Don't forget to exercise today.

Snack

A peach (42 calories)

Dinner

Sashimi appetizer (2 pieces, 164 calories)
Honey orange glazed salmon (390 calories)
Stir fried vegetables
A glass of red wine (3½ ounces, 74 calories)
Iced green tea

Snack

Roasted plums

Sunday, week 2, breakfast

Low fat whole grain waffles with low calorie strawberry syrup (three 4" waffles, 249 calories, and 3 tablespoons syrup, 75 calories)
6 sliced strawberries (24 calories)
A glass of orange juice (110 calories)
If desired, a cup of coffee with skim milk and flavored with NutraSweet

Snack

Tropical fruit salad: diced mango, papaya, and kiwi (210 calories)

Lunch

Nicoise salad: tuna atop mixed greens, 4 green beans, 1 sliced baby potato, diced egg white, and 2 black olives (300 calories)
A peach (42 calories)
Water with lemon

Snack

10 grapes (36 calories)

Dinner

Gazpacho with shrimp (60 calories)
Eye of round roast, fat cut away (6 ounces, 286 calories)
Sautéed onions and mushrooms
Baked sweet potatoes (150 calories)
Green peas with rosemary and diced red pepper (½ cup, 116 calories)
A glass of red wine (3½ ounces, 74 calories)
Water

Snack

A piece of angel food cake (129 calories) with ½ sliced peach sprinkled with cinnamon

Monday, week 2, breakfast

Raisin bran cereal (1 cup, 186 calories) with skim milk (½ cup, 43 calories)
A glass of skim milk (86 calories)
Orange banana smoothie with vanilla nonfat yogurt (206 calories)
If desired a cup of coffee with skim milk and flavored with NutraSweet

Try to go running today.

Snack

4 tablespoons of roasted red pepper hummus (92 calories) and 8 baby carrots (32 calories)
2 dried figs (97 calories)

Lunch

1 ounce nonfat cream cheese, basil, tomato, and red onion on low calorie bread (248 calories)
Cucumber dill salad
Lemonade sweetened with NutraSweet (5 calories)

Snack

Poached pear (150 calories)

Dinner

Chopped vegetable salad (100 calories)
Potato gnocchi with marinara sauce (1 cup, 340 calories)
Puréed squash (¾ cup, 60 calories)
A glass of red wine if desired (3½ ounces, 74 calories)
Water with lemon

Snack

Sugar-free jello (½ cup, 8 calories) with 10 sour cherries (25 calories)

Tuesday, week 2, breakfast

Low fat ricotta-applesauce pancakes with blueberries (248 calories)
A tangerine (37 calories)
A glass of tomato juice (41 calories)
If desired, a cup of coffee with skim milk and flavored with NutraSweet

Go to the gym today.

Snack

Frozen banana (109 calories) coated in crushed macadamia nuts (203 calories)

Lunch

Minestrone soup (1 cup, 82 calories)
3 slices pizza with nonfat mozzarella, mushrooms, and olives (396 calories)
Diet soda (4 calories)

Snack

Nonfat yogurt with fruit (8 ounces, 213 calories).

Dinner

Mixed greens salad with strawberries, toasted pine nuts, and balsamic vinaigrette (95 calories)
Baked fillet of sole pinwheels stuffed with julienned vegetables (224 calories)
Almond rice pilaf (1 cup, 222 calories)
A glass of red wine (3½ ounces, 74 calories)
10 grapes (36 calories)
Water with lemon

Snack

Nonfat vanilla pudding (½ cup, 105 calories)

Wednesday, week 2, breakfast

Muesli cereal "parfait" (⅔ cup, 190 calories) with nonfat vanilla yogurt (½ cup, 44 calories) and sliced banana
A glass of orange juice
4 vegetarian breakfast links (126 calories)
If desired, a cup of coffee with skim milk and flavored with NutraSweet

Go running today.

Snack

Pineapple grilled with lemon and honey (72 calories)
Nonfat cottage cheese (1 cup, 123 calories)

Lunch

Salad topped with crab cake and mango salsa (250 calories)
Water or diet soda

Snack

Almond stuffed dates

Dinner

Butternut squash soup
Skinless turkey breast (6 ounces, 266 calories) with cranberry-apple compote
Mashed potatoes (⅓ cup, 83 calories)
Roasted baby carrots with cumin
A glass of wine if desired (3½ ounces, 74 calories)
Water

Snack

A piece of lemon meringue pie (303 calories)

Thursday, week 2, breakfast

Cream of wheat (1 cup, 133 calories) with raspberries (¾ cup, 45 calories)

A glass of skim milk (86 calories)

If desired a cup of coffee with skim milk and flavored with NutraSweet

Go to the gym today.

Snack

Peanut butter smoothie: 1 tablespoon peanut butter, ½ cup vanilla frozen yogurt, 1 tablespoon sliced almonds, and ⅓ cup nonfat milk

Lunch

Green salad with red onion, cherry tomatoes, and vinaigrette (49 calories)

2 chicken soft tacos with chicken breast, salsa, and low fat sour cream (280 calories)

10 grapes (36 calories)

Snack

2 plums (72 calories)

Nonfat vanilla pudding (4 ounces, 105 calories)

Dinner

Baby spinach salad with nectarines and spiced pecans (75 calories)

Pasta with grilled chicken and vegetable marinara (395 calories)

A glass of red wine (3½ ounces, 74 calories)

Water

Snack

A piece of cherry pie (304 calories)

Friday, week 2, breakfast

Oatmeal (1 cup, 145 calories) with chopped apple, almonds, and cinnamon
A banana (109 calories)
A glass of skim milk (86 calories)
If desired a cup of coffee with skim milk and flavored with NutraSweet

Go running today.

Snack

Cucumber slices topped with baby shrimp (6 ounces, 204 calories)

Lunch

Black bean soup with nonfat sour cream (100 calories)
Tossed salad topped with shrimp, cubed pineapple, watermelon, cucumber, and
bell pepper with lime dressing (218 calories)
Iced tea sweetened with NutraSweet (7 calories)
Water

Snack

2 star fruit or kiwi fruit (60 calories)
12 macadamia nuts (203 calories)

Dinner

Low fat turkey meatloaf (240 calories)
Mashed potatoes made with water or skim milk (1 cup, 162 calories)
Zucchini "pasta" (70 calories)
A glass of wine (3½ ounces, 74 calories)

Snack

Nonfat tapioca pudding (98 calories)

Saturday, week 2, breakfast

2 pancakes prepared from low calorie mix (148 calories) with mixed berries added (1 cup, 60 calories)
Low calorie pancake syrup (2 tablespoons, 50 calories)
A glass of skim milk (86 calories)
If desired a cup of coffee with skim milk and flavored with NutraSweet

Don't forget to exercise today.

Snack

12 macadamia nuts (203 calories)

Lunch

Mixed greens with raspberries and raspberry vinaigrette (43 calories)
2 chicken soft tacos with chicken breast, salsa, and low fat sour cream (280 calories)
Watermelon (one wedge, 92 calories)
Lemonade sweetened with NutraSweet

Snack

An apple (81 calories)

Dinner

Baby spinach and jicama salad with grapefruit segments and cider vinaigrette (130 calories)
Broiled skinless chicken breast with mango salsa (150 calories)
Oven roasted "fries" with herbs (½ baking potato cut into shoestring size) (220 calories)
8 asparagus spears (32 calories)
A glass of red wine (3½ ounces, 74 calories)
Water

Snack

A piece of cherry pie (304 calories)

Sunday, week 3, breakfast

Raisin bran cereal with skim milk (1 cup cereal with ½ cup milk, 229 calories)
2 apricots (34 calories)
A glass of tomato juice (41 calories)
If desired a cup of coffee with skim milk and flavored with NutraSweet

Snack

Honeydew melon or cantaloupe (⅛ melon, 56 calories) with nonfat cottage cheese (123 calories)

Lunch

Couscous chicken salad with garbanzo beans, cherry tomatoes, and basil (322 calories)
10 grapes (36 calories)
Low calorie lemonade
Water

Snack

A peach (42 calories)

Dinner

Baby spinach salad with nectarines, spicy pecans, and balsamic shallot dressing (75 calories)
Sweet and sour tofu with rice (275 calories)
2 sliced cooked carrots (62 calories)
Diet soda or water
A glass of red wine (3½ ounces, 74 calories)

Snack

A piece of blueberry pie (271 calories)

Monday, week 3, breakfast

Peanut butter and jelly sandwich (2 tablespoons natural peanut butter, low calorie jelly, 332 calories) with sliced half banana (55 calories)
A glass of orange juice (112 calories)
If desired a cup of coffee with skim milk and flavored with NutraSweet

Go running today.

Snack

Nonfat yogurt with fruit (8 ounces, 213 calories)

Lunch

Mixed lettuce with crabmeat salad (191 calories) with 2 slices avocado and cherry tomatoes
An apple (81 calories)
Diet soda, tea, or coffee
Water

Snack

Sliced apple with cinnamon (81 calories) and vanilla yogurt dip

Dinner

Poached salmon with julienned vegetables (400 calories)
Lentil salad (180 calories)
A glass of wine if desired (3½ ounces, 74 calories)
Water

Snack

2 baked plums (72 calories)

Tuesday, week 3, breakfast

2 slices of French toast made with egg substitute (252 calories), cinnamon-orange zest, and vanilla
Low calorie syrup (2 tablespoons, 50 calories)
Citrus salad: mixed grapefruit, orange, and tangerine segments with lime juice and chopped mint (150 calories)
Orange juice (1 cup, 112 calories)
If desired a cup of coffee with skim milk and flavored with NutraSweet

Go to the gym today.

Snack

Shrimp cocktail (5 shrimps with cocktail sauce, 100 calories)

Lunch

1 ounce nonfat cream cheese, basil, tomato, and red onion on low calorie bread (248 calories)
Cucumber-dill salad (40 calories)
2 dried figs (97 calories)
Diet soda, tea, or coffee (5 calories)
Water

Snack

28 peanuts (166 calories)
10 grapes (36 calories)

Dinner

Carrot ginger soup (120 calories)
Mixed mushroom/roasted red pepper lasagna with nonfat mozzarella and Parmesan cheese (400 calories)
A glass of red wine (3½ ounces, 74 calories)
Water

Snack

Summer fruit soup (185 calories)

Wednesday, week 3, breakfast

Cream of wheat cereal (1 cup, 133 calories) with 6 sliced strawberries (24 calories)

A glass of skim milk (86 calories)

If desired a cup of coffee with skim milk and flavored with NutraSweet

Go running today.

Snack

Frozen banana (109 calories) rolled in crushed macadamias (203 calories)

Lunch

Garden salad with 2 tablespoons low calorie dressing (65 calories)

Two Morningstar Farms Meatless Griller patties topped with a slice of nonfat cheese and sliced tomato (342 calories)

2 tablespoons ketchup (32 calories)

Diet soda, tea, or coffee

Water

Snack

Nonfat yogurt with NutraSweet (98 calories)

Dinner

Spice crusted salmon with nonfat yogurt sour cream citrus sauce (308 calories)

Green beans and sliced toasted almonds with Dijon mustard and lemon vinaigrette (54 calories)

Rice (1 cup, 205 calories)

A glass of wine if desired (3½ ounces, 74 calories)

Diet soda or water

Snack

A piece of lemon meringue pie (303 calories)

Thursday, week 3, breakfast

Omelette with egg substitute (¾ cup, 159 calories) or egg whites, three slices of nonfat cheese (93 calories), and a few slices of avocado
A glass of skim milk (86 calories)
8 strawberries (32 calories)
If desired a cup of coffee with skim milk and flavored with NutraSweet

Go to the gym today.

Snack

½ cup roasted red pepper-olive hummus with vegetable sticks and ½ whole wheat pita (250 calories)
5 black olives (25 calories)
Cucumber slices (10 calories)

Lunch

Japanese soba noodle salad with snow peas, carrots, peas, mushrooms, and scallion (310 calories) with tofu
Iced green tea
Diet soda
Water with lime

Snack

12 macadamia nuts (203 calories)
Nonfat chocolate pudding (4 ounces, 107 calories)

Dinner

Orange, tomato, and jicama salad (82 calories)
Cheeseless lasagna with tomato, zucchini, basil, and red bell pepper sauce (382 calories)
A glass of red wine (3½ ounces, 74 calories)
Water
A plum (36 calories)

Snack

A piece of blueberry pie (271 calories)

Friday, week 3, breakfast

3 low fat wild rice pancakes (220 calories)
Date-nut smoothie with nonfat yogurt
If desired, a cup of coffee with skim milk and flavored with NutraSweet

Go running today.

Snack

Grilled fruit skewers with nonfat vanilla yogurt

Lunch

Tossed salad with 2 tablespoons low calorie dressing (65 calories)
3 slices pizza with nonfat mozzarella, mushrooms, and olives (396 calories)
2 plums (72 calories)
Diet soda, coffee, or tea
Water

Snack

Banana half spread with peanut butter and topped with 14 chopped peanuts (190 calories)

Dinner

Corn chowder (135 calories)
Baked red snapper with tomato, olives, and capers (235 calories)
Herb roasted red potatoes (214 calories)
A glass of wine (3½ ounces, 74 calories)
Water

Snack

Nonfat vanilla pudding (½ cup, 105 calories)

Saturday, week 3, breakfast

Scrambled egg substitute (¾ cup, 159 calories) or egg white omelette with rata-
touille (91 calories)
A banana (109 calories)
A glass of skim milk (86 calories)
If desired a cup of coffee with skim milk and flavored with NutraSweet

Snack

Eggplant dip with celery sticks

Lunch

A can of light tuna with mixed in nonfat mayonnaise, chopped scallion, dill,
celery, lemon juice stuffed into 2 tomato halves (410 calories)
Watermelon (1 wedge, 92 calories)
Iced tea sweetened with NutraSweet
Water with lemon

Snack

Mixed berries

Dinner

Grilled vegetable antipasto (122 calories)
Grilled sirloin steak fat cut away (6 ounces, 332 calories) with roasted red pep-
per sauce (2 tablespoons, 25 calories)
Cider roasted beets, carrots, and parsnips (157 calories)
A glass of red wine (3½ ounces, 74 calories)
Water

Snack

A piece of blueberry pie (271 calories)

References

1 Kant AK, Graubard BI. Energy density of diets reported by American adults: association with food group intake, nutrient intake, and body weight. *Int J Obes Relat Metab Disord.* 2005 Aug;29(8):95.

2 Potter, J, ed. *Food, Nutrition and the Prevention of Cancer: a global perspective.* Washington: World Cancer Research Fund, 1997.

3 Third Report of the National Cholesterol Education Program (NCEP) Expert Panel on Detection, Evaluation, and Treatment of High Blood Cholesterol in Adults (Adult Treatment Panel III) final report. *Circulation.* 2002 Dec 17;106(25):3143-421.

4 Stampfer MJ, Hu FB, Manson JE, Rimm EB, Willett WC. Primary prevention of coronary heart disease in women through diet and lifestyle. *N Engl J Med.* 2000 Jul 6;343(1):16-22.

5 Sempos CT, Cleeman JI, Carroll MD, Johnson CL, Bachorik PS, Gordon DJ, Burt VL, Briefel RR, Brown CD, Lippel K, et al. Prevalence of high blood cholesterol among US adults. An update based on guidelines from the second report of the National Cholesterol Education Program Adult Treatment Panel. JAMA. 1993 Jun 16;269(23):3009-14.

6 Stamler J, Wentworth D, Neaton JD. Is relationship between serum cholesterol and risk of premature death from coronary heart disease continuous and graded? Findings in 356,222 primary screenees of the Multiple Risk Factor Intervention Trial (MRFIT). JAMA. 1986 Nov 28;256(20):2823-8.

7 Kushi L, Giovannucci E. Dietary fat and cancer. *Am J Med.* 2002 Dec 30;113 Suppl 9B:63S-70S.

8 Poschl G, Seitz HK. Alcohol and cancer. *Alcohol.* 2004 May-Jun;39(3):155-65.

9 McCullough ML, Giovannucci EL. Diet and cancer prevention. *Oncogene.* 2004 Aug 23;23(38):6349-64.

10 Key TJ, Allen NE, Spencer EA, Travis RC. Nutrition and breast cancer. *Breast.* 2003 Dec;12(6):412-6.

11 Tsukada K, Miyazaki T, Kato H, Masuda N, Fukuchi M, Fukai Y, Nakajima M, Ishizaki M, Motegi M, Mogi A, Sohda M, Moteki T, Sekine T, Kuwano H. Body fat accumulation and postoperative complications after abdominal surgery. *Am Surg.* 2004 Apr;70(4):347-51.

12 Hoffmann R. The thrombo-embolic risk in surgery. *Hepatogastroenterology.* 1991 Aug;38(4):272-8.

13 *Wall Street Journal,* February 10, 2004.

14 National Health and Nutrition Examination Survey, 2000.

15 Atkins RC. *Dr. Atkins' New Diet Revolution.* 3rd ed. Avon, 2001.

16 Barry Sears, Bill Lawren. *The Zone: A Dietary Road Map to Lose Weight Permanently: Reset Your Generic Code: Prevent Disease: Achieve Maximum Physical Performance.* ReganBooks, 1995.

17 Atkins RC. *Dr. Atkins' New Diet Revolution.* 3rd ed. Avon, 2001, p. 58-65.

18 Astrup A, Ryan L, Grunwald GK, Storgaard M, Saris W, Melanson E, Hill JO. The role of dietary fat in body fatness: evidence from a preliminary meta-analysis of ad libitum low-fat dietary intervention studies. *Br J Nutr.* 2000 Mar;83 Suppl 1:S25-32.

19 Katz DL. Pandemic obesity and the contagion of nutritional nonsense. *Public Health Rev.* 2003;31(1):33-44.

20 Keys A. *Seven Countries: A multivariate analysis of death and coronary heart disease.* Cambridge, MA: Harvard University Press, 1980.

21 Hu FB, Manson JE, Willett WC. Types of dietary fat and risk of coronary heart disease: a critical review. *J Am Coll Nutr.* 2001 Feb;20(1):5-19.

22 Anderson JW, Konz EC, Jenkins DJ. Health advantages and disadvantages of weight-reducing diets: a computer analysis and critical review. *J Am Coll Nutr.* 2000 Oct;19(5):578-90.

23 Ornish D, Scherwitz LW, Billings JH, Brown SE, Gould KL, Merritt TA, Sparler S, Armstrong WT, Ports TA, Kirkeeide RL, Hogeboom C, Brand RJ. Intensive lifestyle changes for reversal of coronary heart disease. JAMA. 1998 Dec 16;280(23):2001-7.

24 Agatston A. *The South Beach Diet*. New York: Random House, 2003.

25 Raben A. Should obese patients be counselled to follow a low-glycaemic index diet? No. *Obes Rev*. 2002 Nov;3(4):245-56.

26 Beyer PL, Flynn MA. Effects of high- and low-fiber diets on human feces. *J Am Diet Assoc*. 1978 Mar;72(3):271-7.

27 Scrimshaw NS. The phenomenon of famine. *Annu Rev Nutr*. 1987;7:1-21.

28 *New York* magazine, June 30, 2003.

29 Brousseau ME, Schaefer EJ. Diet and coronary heart disease: clinical trials. *Curr Atheroscler Rep*. 2000 Nov;2(6):487-93.

30 *Good Morning America*, October 26, 2004

31 Moore JG, Christian PE, Coleman RE. Gastric emptying of varying meal weight and composition in man. Evaluation by dual liquid- and solid-phase isotopic method. *Dig Dis Sci*. 1981 Jan;26(1):16-22.

32 Feinle C. Role of intestinal chemoreception in the induction of gastrointestinal sensations. *Dtsch Tierarztl Wochenschr*. 1998 Dec;105(12):441-4.

33 Manson JE, Willett WC, Stampfer MJ, Colditz GA, Hunter DJ, Hankinson SE, Hennekens CH, Speizer FE. Body weight and mortality among women. *N Engl J Med*. 1995;333:677-685.

34 Rabkin SW, Mathewson FA, Hsu PH. Relation of body weight to development of ischemic heart disease in a cohort of young North American men after a 26 year observation period: the Manitoba Study. *Am J Cardiol*. 1977;39:452-458.

35 Vainio H, Bianchini F. *IARC handbooks of cancer prevention. Volume 6: Weight control and physical activity*. Lyon, France: IARC Press, 2002.

36 National Health and Nutrition Examination Survey, 1988-1994.

37 Colditz GA, Willett WC, Rotnitzky A, Manson JE. Weight gain as a risk factor for clinical diabetes mellitus in women. *Ann Intern Med*. 1995 Apr 1;122(7):481-6.

38 Allison DB, Fontaine KR, Manson JE, Stevens J, VanItallie TB. Annual deaths attributable to obesity in the United States. JAMA 1999.

39 Manson JE, Willett WC, Stampfer MJ, Colditz GA, Hunter DJ, Hankinson SE, Hennekens CH, Speizer FE. Body weight and mortality in women. *N Engl J Med* 1995;333:677-685.

40 Solomon CG, Manson JE. Obesity and mortality: a review of the epidemiologic data. *Am J Clin Nutr*. 1997 Oct;66(4 Suppl):1044S-1050S.

41 Peeters A, Barendregt JJ, Willekens F, Mackenbach JP, Al Mamun A, Bonneux L. Obesity in Adulthood and Its Consequences for Life Expectancy: A Life-Table Analysis. *Ann Int Medicine*. 2003; 138: 24-32.

42 Fontaine KR, Redden DT, Wang C, Westfall AO, Allison DB. Years of life lost due to obesity. JAMA. 2003 Jan 8;289(2):187-93.

43 Rexrode KM, Manson JE, Hennekens CH. Obesity and cardiovascular disease. *Curr Opin Cardiol*. 1996 Sep;11(5):490-5.

44 Key TJ, Schatzkin A, Willett WC, Allen NE, Spencer EA, Travis RC. Diet, nutrition and the prevention of cancer. *Public Health Nutr*. 2004 Feb;7(1A):187-200.

45 Mayer CE, Joyce A. The Escalating Obesity Wars: Nonprofit's Tactics, Funding Sources Spark Controversy. *Washington Post*. 2005 April 27; E01.

46 Tovee MJ, Maisey DS, Emery JL, Cornelissen PL. Visual cues to female physical attractiveness.*Proc R Soc Lond B Biol Sci*. 1999 Jan 22;266(1415):211-8.

47 Clayson DE, Klassen ML. Perception of attractiveness by obesity and hair color. *Percept Mot Skills*. 1989 Feb;68(1):199-202.

48 Janssen I, Craig WM, Boyce WF, Pickett W. Associations between overweight and obesity with bullying behaviors in school-aged children. *Pediatrics*. 2004 May;113(5):1187-94.

49 Roehling M. Weight-Based Discrimination in Employment: Psychological and Legal Aspects. *Personnel Psychology*. 1999; 52: 969-1016.

50 Sutcliffe JF. A review of in vivo experimental methods to determine the composition of the human body. *Phys Med Biol*. 1996 May;41(5):791-833.

51 Hannan WJ, Wrate RM, Cowen SJ, Freeman CP. Body mass index as an estimate of body fat. *Int J Eat Disord*. 1995 Jul;18(1):91-7.

52 Lean ME, Han TS, Seidell JC. Impairment of health and quality of life in people with large waist circumference. *Lancet*. 1998 Mar 21;351(9106):853-6.

53 Mann JI. Diet and risk of coronary heart disease and type 2 diabetes. *Lancet*. 2002 Sep 7;360(9335):783-9.

54 Hu FB, Manson JE, Willett WC. Types of dietary fat and risk of coronary heart disease: a critical review. *J Am Coll Nutr*. 2001 Feb;20(1):5-19.

55 Harper CR, Jacobson TA. Beyond the Mediterranean diet: the role of omega-3 Fatty acids in the prevention of coronary heart disease. *Prev Cardiol*. 2003 Summer;6(3):136-46.

56 Hu FB, Bronner L, Willett WC, Stampfer MJ, Rexrode KM, Albert CM, Hunter D, Manson JE. Fish and omega-3 fatty acid intake and risk of coronary heart disease in women. JAMA. 2002 Apr 10;287(14):1815-21.

57 Marckmann P, Gronbaek M. Fish consumption and coronary heart disease mortality. A systematic review of prospective cohort studies. *Eur J Clin Nutr*. 1999 Aug;53(8):585-90.

58 Hu FB, Stampfer MJ. Nut consumption and risk of coronary heart disease: a review of epidemiologic evidence. *Curr Atheroscler Rep*. 1999 Nov;1(3):204-9.

59 Lukito W. Candidate foods in the asia-pacific region for cardiovascular protection: nuts, soy, lentils and tempe. *Asia Pac J Clin Nutr*. 2001;10(2):128-33.

60 Hunter JE. n-3 fatty acids from vegetable oils. *Am J Clin Nutr*. 1990 May;51(5):809-14.

61 Cunnane SC, Ganguli S, Menard C, Liede AC, Hamadeh MJ, Chen ZY, Wolever TM, Jenkins DJ. High alpha-linolenic acid flaxseed (Linum usitatissimum): some nutritional properties in humans. *Br J Nutr*. 1993 Mar;69(2):443-53.

62 Osterud B, Bjorklid E. Role of monocytes in atherogenesis. *Physiol Rev*. 2003 Oct;83(4):1069-112.

63 Sacks FM, Katan M. Randomized clinical trials on the effects of dietary fat and carbohydrate on plasma lipoproteins and cardiovascular disease. *Am J Med*. 2002 Dec 30;113 Suppl 9B:13S-24S.

64 National Cholesterol Education Program (NCEP) Expert Panel on Detection, Evaluation, and Treatment of High Blood Cholesterol in Adults (Adult Treatment Panel III). Third Report of the National Cholesterol Education Program (NCEP) Expert Panel on Detection, Evaluation, and Treatment of High Blood Cholesterol in Adults (Adult Treatment Panel III) final report. Circulation. 2002 Dec 17;106(25):3143-421.

65 National Cholesterol Education Program (NCEP) Expert Panel on Detection, Evaluation, and Treatment of High Blood Cholesterol in Adults (Adult Treatment Panel III). Third Report of the National Cholesterol Education Program (NCEP) Expert Panel on Detection, Evaluation, and Treatment of High Blood Cholesterol in Adults (Adult Treatment Panel III) final report. *Circulation*. 2002 Dec 17;106(25):3143-421.

66 LaRosa JC. New and emerging data from clinical trials of statins. *Curr Atheroscler Rep*. 2004 Jan;6(1):12-9.

67 National Cholesterol Education Program (NCEP) Expert Panel on Detection, Evaluation, and Treatment of High Blood Cholesterol in Adults (Adult Treatment Panel III). Third Report of the National Cholesterol Education Program (NCEP) Expert Panel on Detection, Evaluation, and Treatment of High Blood Cholesterol in Adults (Adult Treatment Panel III) final report. Circulation. 2002 Dec 17;106(25):3143-421.

68 Spieker LE, Ruschitzka F, Luscher TF, Noll G. HDL and inflammation in atherosclerosis. *Curr Drug Targets Immune Endocr Metabol Disord*. 2004 Mar;4(1):51-7.

69 Navab M, Hama SY, Cooke CJ, Anantharamaiah GM, Chaddha M, Jin L, Subbanagounder G, Faull KF, Reddy ST, Miller NE, Fogelman AM. Normal high density lipoprotein inhibits three steps in the formation of mildly oxidized low density lipoprotein: step 1. *J Lipid Res*. 2000 Sep;41(9):1481-94.

70 Navab M, Hama SY, Anantharamaiah GM, Hassan K, Hough GP, Watson AD, Reddy ST, Sevanian A, Fonarow GC, Fogelman AM. Normal high density lipoprotein inhibits three steps in the formation of mildly oxidized low density lipoprotein: steps 2 and 3. *J Lipid Res*. 2000 Sep;41(9):1495-508.

71 Wilson PWF, D'Agostino RB, Levy D, Belanger AM, Silbershatz H, Kannel WB. Prediction of coronary heart disease using risk factor categories. *Circulation* 1998;97:1837-47.

72 Brown CD, Higgins M, Donato KA, Rohde FC, Garrison R, Obarzanek E, Ernst ND, Horan M. Body mass index and the prevalence of hypertension and dyslipidemia. *Obes Res.* 2000 Dec;8(9):605-19.

73 Szapary PO, Bloedon LT, Foster GD. Physical activity and its effects on lipids. *Curr Cardiol Rep.* 2003 Nov;5(6):488-92.

74 Maeda K, Noguchi Y, Fukui T. The effects of cessation from cigarette smoking on the lipid and lipoprotein profiles: a meta-analysis. *Prev Med.* 2003 Oct;37(4):283-90.

75 Kushi L, Giovannucci E. Dietary fat and cancer. *Am J Med.* 2002 Dec 30;113 Suppl 9B:63S-70S.

76 Jequier E, Bray GA. Low-fat diets are preferred. *Am J Med.* 2002 Dec 30;113 Suppl 9B:41S-46S.

77 Sommerfeld M. Trans unsaturated fatty acids in natural products and processed foods. *Prog Lipid Res.* 1983;22(3):221-33.

78 Sacks FM, Katan M. Randomized clinical trials on the effects of dietary fat and carbohydrate on plasma lipoproteins and cardiovascular disease. *Am J Med.* 2002 Dec 30;113 Suppl 9B:13S-24S.

79 Ascherio A, Hennekens CH, Buring JE, Master C, Stampfer MJ, Willett WC. Trans fatty acids intake and risk of myocardial infarction. *Circulation* 1994; 89:94-101.

80 Ascherio A, Rimm EB, Giovannucci EL, Spiegelman D, Stampfer MJ, Willett WC. Dietary fat and risk of coronary heart disease in men: cohort follow up study in the United States. *BMJ* 1996; 313:84-90.

81 Pietinen P, Ascherio A, Korhonen P, et al. Intake of fatty acids and risk of coronary heart disease in a cohort of Finnish men: The ATBC Study. *Am J Epidemiol* 1997; 145:876-887.

82 Hu FB, Stampfer MJ, Manson JE, et al. Dietary fat intake and the risk of coronary heart disease in women. *N Engl J Med* 1997; 337:1491-1499.

83 Food and Drug Administration, HHS. Food labeling: trans fatty acids in nutrition labeling, nutrient content claims, and health claims. Final rule. *Fed Regist.* 2003 Jul 11;68(133):41433-1506.

84 Snowdon DA, Phillips RL, Fraser GE. Meat consumption and fatal ischemic heart disease. *Prev Med.* 1984 Sep;13(5):490-500.

85 Wei EK, Giovannucci E, Wu K, Rosner B, Fuchs CS, Willett WC, Colditz GA. Comparison of risk factors for colon and rectal cancer. *Int J Cancer.* 2004 Jan 20;108(3):433-42.

86 Giovannucci E. Diet, body weight, and colorectal cancer: a summary of the epidemiologic evidence. *J Womens Health (Larchmt).* 2003 Mar;12(2):173-82.

87 Ferguson LR. Natural and human-made mutagens and carcinogens in the human diet. *Toxicology.* 2002 Dec 27;181-182:79-82.

88 European Commission Health and Consumer Protection Directorate-General Scientific Committee on Food, Polycyclic aromatic hydrocarbons—occurrence in foods, dietary exposure and health effects, 2002.

89 Le Marchand L, Hankin JH, Pierce LM, Sinha R, Nerurkar PV, Franke AA, Wilkens LR, Kolonel LN, Donlon T, Seifried A, Custer LJ, Lum-Jones A, Chang W. Well-done red meat, metabolic phenotypes and colorectal cancer in Hawaii. *Mutat Res.* 2002 Sep 30;506-507:205-14.

90 Sinha R, Rothman N. Role of well-done, grilled red meat, heterocyclic amines (HCAs) in the etiology of human cancer. *Cancer Lett.* 1999 Sep 1;143(2):189-94.

91 Lijinsky W. The formation and occurrence of polynuclear aromatic hydrocarbons associated with food. *Mutat Res.* 1991 Mar-Apr;259(3-4):251-61.

92 European Commission Health and Consumer Protection Directorate-General Scientific Committee on Food, Polycyclic aromatic hydrocarbons—occurrence in foods, dietary exposure and health effects, 2002.

93 ACS News website, ACS Expert Offers Tips on Healthy Holiday Grilling, 2000.

94 Knize MG, Salmon CP, Mehta SS, Felton JS. Analysis of cooked muscle meats for heterocyclic aromatic amine carcinogens. *Mutat Res.* 1997 May 12;376(1-2):129-34.

95 Salmon CP, Knize MG, Felton JS. Effects of marinating on heterocyclic amine carcinogen formation in grilled chicken. *Food Chem Toxicol.* 1997 May;35(5):433-41.

96 Key TJ, Schatzkin A, Willett WC, Allen NE, Spencer EA, Travis RC. Diet, nutrition and the prevention of cancer. *Public Health Nutr.* 2004 Feb;7(1A):187-200.

97 McKnight GM, Duncan CW, Leifert C, Golden MH. Dietary nitrate in man: friend or foe? *Br J Nutr.* 1999 May;81(5):349-58.

98 Eichholzer M, Gutzwiller F. Dietary nitrates, nitrites, and N-nitroso compounds and cancer risk: a review of the epidemiologic evidence. *Nutr Rev.* 1998 Apr;56(4 Pt 1):95-105.

99 Cantor KP. Drinking water and cancer. *Cancer Causes Control.* 1997 May;8(3):292-308.

100 Bang HO, Dyerberg J, Sinclair HM. The composition of the Eskimo food in north western Greenland. *Am J Clin Nutr.* 1980 Dec;33(12):2657-61.

101 Kris-Etherton PM, Harris WS, Appel LJ; American Heart Association. Nutrition Committee. Fish consumption, fish oil, omega-3 fatty acids, and cardiovascular disease. *Circulation.* 2002 Nov 19;106(21):2747-57.

102 Nriagu J, Becker C. Volcanic emissions of mercury to the atmosphere: global and regional inventories. *Sci Total Environ.* 2003 Mar 20;304(1-3):3-12.

103 Jarup L. Hazards of heavy metal contamination. *Br Med Bull.* 2003;68:167-82.

104 Environmental Protection Agency. Mercury Update: Impact on Fish Advisories. June, 2001.

105 Harada M. Minamata disease: methylmercury poisoning in Japan caused by environmental pollution. *Crit Rev Toxicol.* 1995;25(1):1-24.

106 Consumer Advisory. Center for Food Safety and Applied Nutrition, U.S. Food and Drug Administration, 2001.

107 Din JN, Newby DE, Flapan AD. Omega 3 fatty acids and cardiovascular disease—fishing for a natural treatment. *BMJ.* 2004 Jan 3;328(7430):30-5.

108 Marckmann P, Gronbaek M. Fish consumption and coronary heart disease mortality. A systematic review of prospective cohort studies. *Eur J Clin Nutr.* 1999 Aug;53(8):585-90.

109 FDA Surveys 1990-2003.

110 "National Marine Fisheries Service Survey of Trace Elements in the Fishery Resource" Report 1978.

111 "The Occurrence of Mercury in the Fishery Resources of the Gulf of Mexico" Report 2000.

112 Silberhorn EM, Glauert HP, Robertson LW. Carcinogenicity of polyhalogenated biphenyls: PCBs and PBBs. *Crit Rev Toxicol.* 1990;20(6):440-96.

113 Kimbrough RD, Krouskas CA. Human exposure to polychlorinated biphenyls and health effects : a critical synopsis. *Toxicol Rev.* 2003;22(4):217-33.

114 Bosetti C, Negri E, Fattore E, La Vecchia C. Occupational exposure to polychlorinated biphenyls and cancer risk. *Eur J Cancer Prev.* 2003 Aug;12(4):251-5.

115 Daly H, Darvill T, Lonky E, Reihman J, Sargent D. Behavioral effects of prenatal and adult exposure to toxic chemicals found in Lake Ontario fish: two methodological approaches. *Toxicol Ind Health.* 1996 May-Aug;12(3-4):419-26.

116 Hites RA, Foran JA, Carpenter DO, Hamilton MC, Knuth BA, Schwager SJ. Global assessment of organic contaminants in farmed salmon. *Science.* 2004 Jan 9;303(5655):226-9.

117 Trowell H. Definition of dietary fiber and hypotheses that it is a protective factor in certain diseases. *Am J Clin Nutr.* 1976 Apr;29(4):417-27.

118 Fernandez ML. Soluble fiber and nondigestible carbohydrate effects on plasma lipids and cardiovascular risk. *Curr Opin Lipidol.* 2001 Feb;12(1):35-40.

119 Wolk A, Manson JE, Stampfer MJ, Colditz GA, Hu FB, Speizer FE, Hennekens CH, Willett WC. Long-term intake of dietary fiber and decreased risk of coronary heart disease among women. *JAMA.* 1999 Jun 2;281(21):1998-2004.

120 Bazzano LA, He J, Ogden LG, Loria CM, Whelton PK. Dietary fiber intake and reduced risk of coronary heart disease in US men and women: the National Health and Nutrition Examination Survey I Epidemiologic Follow-up Study. *Arch Intern Med.* 2003 Sep 8;163(16):1897-904.

121 Jenkins DJ, Wolever TM, Rao AV, Hegele RA, Mitchell SJ, Ransom TP, Boctor DL, Spadafora PJ, Jenkins AL, Mehling C, et al. Effect on blood lipids of very high intakes of fiber in diets low in saturated fat and cholesterol. *N Engl J Med.* 1993 Jul 1;329(1):21-6.

122 Li BW, Andrews KW, Pehrsson, PR. Individual sugars, soluble, and insoluble dietary fiber contents of 70 high consumption foods. *J Food Composition and Analysis* (2002) 15, 715-723.
123 USDA 2005 Dietary Guidelines Advisory Committee.
124 Rissanen TH, Voutilainen S, Virtanen JK, Venho B, Vanharanta M, Mursu J, Salonen JT. Low intake of fruits, berries and vegetables is associated with excess mortality in men: the Kuopio Ischaemic Heart Disease Risk Factor (KIHD) Study. *J Nutr.* 2003 Jan;133(1):199-204.
125 Pereira MA, O'Reilly E, Augustsson K, Fraser GE, Goldbourt U, Heitmann BL, Hallmans G, Knekt P, Liu S, Pietinen P, Spiegelman D, Stevens J, Virtamo J, Willett WC, Ascherio A. Dietary fiber and risk of coronary heart disease: a pooled analysis of cohort studies. *Arch Intern Med.* 2004 Feb 23;164(4):370-6.
126 Bingham SA, Day NE, Luben R, Ferrari P, Slimani N, Norat T, Clavel-Chapelon F, Kesse E, Nieters A, Boeing H, Tjonneland A, Overvad K, Martinez C, Dorronsoro M, Gonzalez CA, Key TJ, Trichopoulou A, Naska A, Vineis P, Tumino R, Krogh V, Bueno-de-Mesquita HB, Peeters PH, Berglund G, Hallmans G, Lund E, Skeie G, Kaaks R, Riboli E; European Prospective Investigation into Cancer and Nutrition. Dietary fibre in food and protection against colorectal cancer in the European Prospective Investigation into Cancer and Nutrition (EPIC): an observational study. *Lancet.* 2003 May 3;361(9368):1496-501.
127 Peters U, Sinha R, Chatterjee N, Subar AF, Ziegler RG, Kulldorff M, Bresalier R, Weissfeld JL, Flood A, Schatzkin A, Hayes RB; Prostate, Lung, Colorectal, and Ovarian Cancer Screening Trial Project Team. Dietary fibre and colorectal adenoma in a colorectal cancer early detection programme. *Lancet.* 2003 May 3;361(9368):1491-5.
128 Giovannucci E, Rimm EB, Stampfer MJ, Colditz GA, Ascherio A, Willett WC. Intake of fat, meat, and fiber in relation to risk of colon cancer in men. *Cancer Res.* 1994 May 1;54(9):2390-7.
129 Fuchs CS, Giovannucci EL, Colditz GA, Hunter DJ, Stampfer MJ, Rosner B, Speizer FE, Willett WC. Dietary fiber and the risk of colorectal cancer and adenoma in women. *N Engl J Med.* 1999 Jan 21;340(3):169-76.
130 Larsson SC, Rafter J, Holmberg L, Bergkvist L, Wolk A. Red meat consumption and risk of cancers of the proximal colon, distal colon and rectum: The Swedish Mammography Cohort. *Int J Cancer.* 2005 Feb 20;113(5):829-34.
131 English DR, MacInnis RJ, Hodge AM, Hopper JL, Haydon AM, Giles GG. Red meat, chicken, and fish consumption and risk of colorectal cancer. *Cancer Epidemiol Biomarkers Prev.* 2004 Sep;13(9):1509-14.
132 Norat T, Lukanova A, Ferrari P, Riboli E. Meat consumption and colorectal cancer risk: dose-response meta-analysis of epidemiological studies. *Int J Cancer.* 2002 Mar 10;98(2):241-56.
133 Johnson IT. New approaches to the role of diet in the prevention of cancers of the alimentary tract. *Mutat Res.* 2004 Jul 13;551(1-2):9-28.
134 Terry P, Giovannucci E, Michels KB, Bergkvist L, Hansen H, Holmberg L, Wolk A. Fruit, vegetables, dietary fiber, and risk of colorectal cancer. *J Natl Cancer Inst.* 2001 Apr 4;93(7):525-33.
135 Hung HC, Joshipura KJ, Jiang R, Hu FB, Hunter D, Smith-Warner SA, Colditz GA, Rosner B, Spiegelman D, Willett WC. Fruit and vegetable intake and risk of major chronic disease. *J Natl Cancer Inst.* 2004 Nov 3;96(21):1577-84.
136 Salmeron J, Manson JE, Stampfer MJ, Colditz GA, Wing AL, Willett WC. Dietary fiber, glycemic load, and risk of non-insulin-dependent diabetes mellitus in women. *JAMA.* 1997 Feb 12;277(6):472-7.
137 Salmeron J, Ascherio A, Rimm EB, Colditz GA, Spiegelman D, Jenkins DJ, Stampfer MJ, Wing AL, Willett WC. Dietary fiber, glycemic load, and risk of NIDDM in men. *Diabetes Care.* 1997 Apr;20(4):545-50.
138 Schulze MB, Liu S, Rimm EB, Manson JE, Willett WC, Hu FB. Glycemic index, glycemic load, and dietary fiber intake and incidence of type 2 diabetes in younger and middle-aged women. *Am J Clin Nutr.* 2004 Aug;80(2):348-56.
139 Dukas L, Willett WC, Giovannucci EL. Association between physical activity, fiber intake, and other lifestyle variables and constipation in a study of women. *Am J Gastroenterol.* 2003 Aug;98(8):1790-6.

140 Metcalf A. Anorectal disorders. Five common causes of pain, itching, and bleeding. *Postgrad Med.* 1995 Nov;98(5):81-4, 87-9, 92-4.

141 Aldoori WH, Giovannucci EL, Rockett HR, Sampson L, Rimm EB, Willett WC. A prospective study of dietary fiber types and symptomatic diverticular disease in men. *J Nutr.* 1998 Apr;128(4):714-9.

142 Floch MH, Bina I. The natural history of diverticulitis: fact and theory. *J Clin Gastroenterol.* 2004 May-Jun;38(5 Suppl):S2-7.

143 Jacobs DR Jr, Steffen LM. Nutrients, foods, and dietary patterns as exposures in research: a framework for food synergy. *Am J Clin Nutr.* 2003 Sep;78(3 Suppl):508S-513S.

144 U.S. Department of Agriculture, *Agriculture Fact Book.* 1998.

145 Jacobs DR Jr, Steffen LM. Nutrients, foods, and dietary patterns as exposures in research: a framework for food synergy. *Am J Clin Nutr.* 2003 Sep;78(3 Suppl):508S-513S.

146 Jacobs DR Jr, Steffen LM. Nutrients, foods, and dietary patterns as exposures in research: a framework for food synergy. *Am J Clin Nutr.* 2003 Sep;78(3 Suppl):508S-513S.

147 Liu S, Stampfer MJ, Hu FB, Giovannucci E, Rimm E, Manson JE, Hennekens CH, Willett WC. Whole-grain consumption and risk of coronary heart disease: results from the Nurses' Health Study. *Am J Clin Nutr.* 1999 Sep;70(3):412-9.

148 Jacobs DR Jr, Meyer KA, Kushi LH, Folsom AR. Whole-grain intake may reduce the risk of ischemic heart disease death in postmenopausal women: the Iowa Women's Health Study. *Am J Clin Nutr.* 1998 Aug;68(2):248-57.

149 Jensen MK, Koh-Banerjee P, Hu FB, Franz M, Sampson L, Gronbaek M, Rimm EB. Intakes of whole grains, bran, and germ and the risk of coronary heart disease in men. *Am J Clin Nutr.* 2004 Dec;80(6):1492-9.

150 Liu S, Manson JE, Stampfer MJ, Hu FB, Giovannucci E, Colditz GA, Hennekens CH, Willett WC. A prospective study of whole-grain intake and risk of type 2 diabetes mellitus in US women. *Am J Public Health.* 2000 Sep;90(9):1409-15.

151 Fung TT, Hu FB, Pereira MA, Liu S, Stampfer MJ, Colditz GA, Willett WC. Whole-grain intake and the risk of type 2 diabetes: a prospective study in men. *Am J Clin Nutr.* 2002 Sep;76(3):535-40.

152 Hu FB, Willett WC. Optimal diets for prevention of coronary heart disease. *JAMA.* 2002 Nov 27;288(20):2569-78.

153 Bazzano LA, He J, Ogden LG, Loria CM, Vupputuri S, Myers L, Whelton PK. Fruit and vegetable intake and risk of cardiovascular disease in US adults: the first National Health and Nutrition Examination Survey Epidemiologic Follow-up Study. *Am J Clin Nutr.* 2002 Jul;76(1):93-9.

154 Key TJ, Schatzkin A, Willett WC, Allen NE, Spencer EA, Travis RC. Diet, nutrition and the prevention of cancer. *Public Health Nutr.* 2004 Feb;7(1A):187-200.

155 Hung HC, Joshipura KJ, Jiang R, Hu FB, Hunter D, Smith-Warner SA, Colditz GA, Rosner B, Spiegelman D, Willett WC. Fruit and vegetable intake and risk of major chronic disease. *J Natl Cancer Inst.* 2004 Nov 3;96(21):1577-84.

156 Johnson IT. New approaches to the role of diet in the prevention of cancers of the alimentary tract. *Mutat Res.* 2004 Jul 13;551(1-2):9-28.

157 Cho E, Seddon JM, Rosner B, Willett WC, Hankinson SE. Prospective study of intake of fruits, vegetables, vitamins, and carotenoids and risk of age-related maculopathy. *Arch Ophthalmol.* 2004 Jun;122(6):883-92.

158 Goldberg J, Flowerdew G, Smith E, Brody JA, Tso MO. Factors associated with age-related macular degeneration. An analysis of data from the first National Health and Nutrition Examination Survey. *Am J Epidemiol.* 1988 Oct;128(4):700-10.

159 Brown L, Rimm EB, Seddon JM, Giovannucci EL, Chasan-Taber L, Spiegelman D, Willett WC, Hankinson SE. A prospective study of carotenoid intake and risk of cataract extraction in US men. *Am J Clin Nutr.* 1999 Oct;70(4):517-24.

160 Joshipura KJ, Hu FB, Manson JE, Stampfer MJ, Rimm EB, Speizer FE, Colditz G, Ascherio A, Rosner B, Spiegelman D, Willett WC. The effect of fruit and vegetable intake on risk for coronary heart disease. *Ann Intern Med.* 2001 Jun 19;134(12):1106-14.

161 Rissanen TH, Voutilainen S, Virtanen JK, Venho B, Vanharanta M, Mursu J, Salonen JT. Low intake of fruits, berries and vegetables is associated with excess mortality in men: the Kuopio Ischaemic Heart Disease Risk Factor (KIHD) Study. J Nutr. 2003 Jan;133(1):199-204.

162 Hu FB, Stampfer MJ, Manson JE, Rimm EB, Colditz GA, Rosner BA, Speizer FE, Hennekens CH, Willett WC. Frequent nut consumption and risk of coronary heart disease in women: prospective cohort study. BMJ. 1998 Nov 14;317(7169):1341-5.

163 Fraser GE, Lindsted KD, Beeson WL. Effect of risk factor values on lifetime risk of and age at first coronary event. The Adventist Health Study. Am J Epidemiol. 1995 Oct 1;142(7):746-58.

164 McCarron DA. The dietary guideline for sodium: should we shake it up? Yes! Am J Clin Nutr. 2000 May;71(5):1013-9.

165 Dahl LK. Possible role of salt intake in the development of essential hypertension. In: Bock KD, Cottier PT, eds. Essential hypertension. Berlin: Springer-Verlag, 1960:53.

166 US Department of Health, Education, and Welfare. Healthy people: Surgeon General's report on health promotion and disease prevention. Washington, DC: US Government Printing Office, 1979.

167 Luft FC, Weinberger MH. Heterogeneous responses to changes in dietary salt intake: the salt-sensitivity paradigm. Am J Clin Nutr. 1997 Feb;65(2 Suppl):612S-617S.

168 Intersalt: an international study of electrolyte excretion and blood pressure. Results for 24 hour urinary sodium and potassium excretion. Intersalt Cooperative Research Group. BMJ. 1988 Jul 30;297(6644):319-28.

169 Midgley JP, Matthew AG, Greenwood CM, Logan AG. Effect of reduced dietary sodium on blood pressure: a meta-analysis of randomized controlled trials. JAMA. 1996 May 22-29;275(20):1590-7.

170 Cutler JA, Follmann D, Allender PS. Randomized trials of sodium reduction: an overview. Am J Clin Nutr. 1997 Feb;65(2 Suppl):643S-651S.

171 Graudal NA, Galloe AM, Garred P. Effects of sodium restriction on blood pressure, renin, aldosterone, catecholamines, cholesterols, and triglyceride: a meta-analysis. JAMA. 1998 May 6;279(17):1383-91.

172 Alderman MH, Cohen H, Madhavan S. Dietary sodium intake and mortality: the National Health and Nutrition Examination Survey (NHANES I). Lancet. 1998 Mar 14;351(9105):781-5.

173 Gruchow HW, Sobocinski KA, Barboriak JJ. Calcium intake and the relationship of dietary sodium and potassium to blood pressure. Am J Clin Nutr. 1988 Dec;48(6):1463-70.

174 Sullivan JM, Prewitt RL, Ratts TE, Josephs JA, Connor MJ. Hemodynamic characteristics of sodium-sensitive human subjects. Hypertension. 1987 Apr;9(4):398-406.

175 Appel LJ, Moore TJ, Obarzanek E, Vollmer WM, Svetkey LP, Sacks FM, Bray GA, Vogt TM, Cutler JA, Windhauser MM, Lin PH, Karanja N. A clinical trial of the effects of dietary patterns on blood pressure. DASH Collaborative Research Group. N Engl J Med. 1997 Apr 17;336(16):1117-24.

176 Joossens JV, Hill MJ, Elliott P, Stamler R, Lesaffre E, Dyer A, Nichols R, Kesteloot H. Dietary salt, nitrate and stomach cancer mortality in 24 countries. European Cancer Prevention (ECP) and the INTERSALT Cooperative Research Group. Int J Epidemiol. 1996 Jun;25(3):494-504.

177 Ngoan LT, Mizoue T, Fujino Y, Tokui N, Yoshimura T. Dietary factors and stomach cancer mortality. Br J Cancer. 2002 Jul 1;87(1):37-42.

178 Key TJ, Schatzkin A, Willett WC, Allen NE, Spencer EA, Travis RC. Diet, nutrition and the prevention of cancer. Public Health Nutr. 2004 Feb;7(1A):187-200.

179 Lind J. A Treatise on Scurvy. 1754.

180 Russell RM. The vitamin A spectrum: from deficiency to toxicity. Am J Clin Nutr. 2000 Apr;71(4):878-84.

181 Dawson EB, Evans DR, Conway ME, McGanity WJ. Vitamin B12 and folate bioavailability from two prenatal multivitamin/multimineral supplements. Am J Perinatol. 2000;17(4):193-9.

182 Dawson EB, Evans DR, McGanity WJ, Conway ME, Harrison DD, Torres-Cantu FM. Bioavailability of iron in two prenatal multivitamin/multimineral supplements. J Reprod Med. 2000 May;45(5):403-9.

183 Srinivasan VS. Bioavailability of nutrients: a practical approach to in vitro demonstration of the availability of nutrients in multivitamin-mineral combination products. *J Nutr.* 2001 Apr;131(4 *Suppl*):1349S-50S.

184 Allen RH, Stabler SP, Savage DG, Lindenbaum J. Metabolic abnormalities in cobalamin (vitamin B12) and folate deficiency. *FASEB J.* 1993 Nov;7(14):1344-53.

185 Kher N, Marsh JD. Pathobiology of atherosclerosis—a brief review. *Semin Thromb Hemost.* 2004 Dec;30(6):665-72.

186 Fruchart JC, Nierman MC, Stroes ES, Kastelein JJ, Duriez P. New risk factors for atherosclerosis and patient risk assessment. *Circulation.* 2004 Jun 15;109(23 Suppl 1):III15-9.

187 Geisel J, Hubner U, Bodis M, Schorr H, Knapp JP, Obeid R, Herrmann W. The role of genetic factors in the development of hyperhomocysteinemia. *Clin Chem Lab Med.* 2003 Nov;41(11):1427-34.

188 Fowler B. Homocysteine: overview of biochemistry, molecular biology, and role in disease processes. *Semin Vasc Med.* 2005 May;5(2):77-86.

189 Carmel R, Green R, Rosenblatt DS, Watkins D. Update on cobalamin, folate, and homocysteine. *Hematology (Am Soc Hematol Educ Program).* 2003; 62-81.

190 Morris MS, Jacques PF, Rosenberg IH, Selhub J, Bowman BA, Gunter EW, Wright JD, Johnson CL. Serum total homocysteine concentration is related to self-reported heart attack or stroke history among men and women in the NHANES III. *J Nutr.* 2000 Dec;130(12):3073-6.

191 Seshadri S, Beiser A, Selhub J, Jacques PF, Rosenberg IH, D'Agostino RB, Wilson PW, Wolf PA. Plasma homocysteine as a risk factor for dementia and Alzheimer's disease. *N Engl J Med.* 2002 Feb 14;346(7):476-83.

192 Ubbink JB. The role of vitamins in the pathogenesis and treatment of hyperhomocyst(e)inaemia. *J Inherit Metab Dis.* 1997 Jun;20(2):316-25.

193 Clarke R, Smith AD, Jobst KA, Refsum H, Sutton L, Ueland PM. Folate, vitamin B12, and serum total homocysteine levels in confirmed Alzheimer disease. *Arch Neurol.* 1998 Nov;55(11):1449-55.

194 Nilsson K, Gustafson L, Hultberg B. Relation between plasma homocysteine and Alzheimer's disease. *Dement Geriatr Cogn Disord.* 2002;14(1):7-12.

195 Luchsinger JA, Tang MX, Shea S, Miller J, Green R, Mayeux R. Plasma homocysteine levels and risk of Alzheimer disease. *Neurology.* 2004 Jun 8;62(11):1972-6.

196 St George-Hyslop PH, Petit A. Molecular biology and genetics of Alzheimer's disease. *C R Biol.* 2005 Feb;328(2):119-30.

197 Luchsinger JA, Tang MX, Shea S, Mayeux R. Caloric intake and the risk of Alzheimer disease. *Arch Neurol.* 2002 Aug;59(8):1258-63.

198 Shekelle P, Hardy ML, Coulter I, Udani J, Spar M, Oda K, Jungvig LK, Tu W, Suttorp MJ, Valentine D, Ramirez L, Shanman R, Newberry SJ. Effect of the supplemental use of antioxidants vitamin C, vitamin E, and coenzyme Q10 for the prevention and treatment of cancer. *Evid Rep Technol Assess (Summ).* 2003 Oct;(75):1-3.

199 Upston JM, Terentis AC, Stocker R. Tocopherol-mediated peroxidation of lipoproteins: implications for vitamin E as a potential antiatherogenic supplement. *FASEB J.* 1999 Jun;13(9):977-94.

200 Rapola JM, Virtamo J, Haukka JK, Heinonen OP, Albanes D, Taylor PR, Huttunen JK. Effect of vitamin E and beta carotene on the incidence of angina pectoris. A randomized, double-blind, controlled trial. *JAMA.* 1996 Mar 6;275(9):693-8.

201 de Gaetano G; Collaborative Group of the Primary Prevention Project. Low-dose aspirin and vitamin E in people at cardiovascular risk: a randomised trial in general practice. Collaborative Group of the Primary Prevention Project. *Lancet.* 2001 Jan 13;357(9250):89-95.

202 Stephens NG, Parsons A, Schofield PM, Kelly F, Cheeseman K, Mitchinson MJ. Randomised controlled trial of vitamin E in patients with coronary disease: Cambridge Heart Antioxidant Study (CHAOS) *Lancet.* 1996 Mar 23;347(9004):781-6.

203 Dietary supplementation with n-3 polyunsaturated fatty acids and vitamin E after myocardial infarction: results of the GISSI-Prevenzione trial. Gruppo Italiano per lo Studio della Sopravvivenza nell'Infarto miocardico. *Lancet.* 1999 Aug 7;354(9177):447-55.

204 Yusuf S, Dagenais G, Pogue J, Bosch J, Sleight P. Vitamin E supplementation and cardiovascular events in high-risk patients. The Heart Outcomes Prevention Evaluation Study Investigators. *N Engl J Med.* 2000 Jan 20;342(3):154-60.

205 Miller ER 3rd, Pastor-Barriuso R, Dalal D, Riemersma RA, Appel LJ, Guallar E. Meta-analysis: high-dosage vitamin E supplementation may increase all-cause mortality. *Ann Intern Med.* 2005 Jan 4;142(1):37-46.

206 Bowry VW, Stocker R. Tocopherol-mediated peroxidation. The prooxidant effect of vitamin E on the radical-initiated oxidation of human low-density lipoprotein. *J. Am. Chem. Soc.* 1993; 115(14):6029-44.

207 Neuzil J, Thomas SR, Stocker R. Requirement for, promotion, or inhibition by alpha-tocopherol of radical-induced initiation of plasma lipoprotein lipid peroxidation. *Free Radic Biol Med.* 1997;22(1-2):57-71.

208 Munteanu A, Zingg JM, Azzi A. Anti-atherosclerotic effects of vitamin E—myth or reality? *J Cell Mol Med.* 2004 Jan-Mar;8(1):59-76.

209 Shekelle P, Hardy ML, Coulter I, Udani J, Spar M, Oda K, Jungvig LK, Tu W, Suttorp MJ, Valentine D, Ramirez L, Shanman R, Newberry SJ. Effect of the supplemental use of antioxidants vitamin C, vitamin E, and coenzyme Q10 for the prevention and treatment of cancer. *Evid Rep Technol Assess (Summ).* 2003 Oct;(75):1-3.

210 Optimal calcium intake. *NIH Consens Statement.* 1994 Jun 6-8;12(4):1-31.

211 Brown AJ, Dusso A, Slatopolsky E. Vitamin D. *Am J Physiol.* 1999 Aug;277(2 Pt 2):F157-75.

212 Prentice A. Diet, nutrition and the prevention of osteoporosis. *Public Health Nutr.* 2004 Feb;7(1A):227-43.

213 Mankin HJ. Rickets, osteomalacia, and renal osteodystrophy. An update. *Orthop Clin North Am.* 1990 Jan;21(1):81-96.

214 Rajakumar K. Vitamin D, cod-liver oil, sunlight, and rickets: a historical perspective. *Pediatrics.* 2003 Aug;112(2):e132-5.

215 Wharton B, Bishop N. Rickets. *Lancet.* 2003 Oct 25;362(9393):1389-400.

216 Vaskonen T. Dietary minerals and modification of cardiovascular risk factors. *J Nutr Biochem.* 2003 Sep;14(9):492-506.

217 Vainio H, Miller AB. Primary and secondary prevention in colorectal cancer. *Acta Oncol.* 2003;42(8):809-15.

218 Standing Committee on the Scientific Evaluation of Dietary Reference Intakes, Food and Nutrition Board, Institute of Medicine, *Dietary Reference Intakes for Calcium, Phosphorus, Magnesium, Vitamin D, and Fluoride,* 1997.

219 Feskanich D, Willett WC, Colditz GA. Calcium, vitamin D, milk consumption, and hip fractures: a prospective study among postmenopausal women. *Am J Clin Nutr.* 2003 Feb;77(2):504-11.

220 Michaelsson K, Melhus H, Bellocco R, Wolk A. Dietary calcium and vitamin D intake in relation to osteoporotic fracture risk. *Bone.* 2003 Jun;32(6):694-703.

221 Rodriguez C, McCullough ML, Mondul AM, Jacobs EJ, Fakhrabadi-Shokoohi D, Giovannucci EL, Thun MJ, Calle EE. Calcium, dairy products, and risk of prostate cancer in a prospective cohort of United States men. *Cancer Epidemiol Biomarkers Prev.* 2003 Jul;12(7):597-603.

222 Chan JM, Stampfer MJ, Ma J, Gann PH, Gaziano JM, Giovannucci EL Dairy products, calcium, and prostate cancer risk in the Physicians' Health Study. *Am J Clin Nutr.* 2001 Oct;74(4):549-54.

223 *Department of Human Services Healthy Guidelines for Americans,* 2000.

224 Mortensen L, Charles P. Bioavailability of calcium supplements and the effect of Vitamin D: comparisons between milk, calcium carbonate, and calcium carbonate plus vitamin D. *Am J Clin Nutr.* 1996 Mar;63(3):354-7.

225 Sheikh MS, Santa Ana CA, Nicar MJ, Schiller LR, Fordtran JS. Gastrointestinal absorption of calcium from milk and calcium salts. *N Engl J Med.* 1987 Aug 27;317(9):532-6.

226 Heaney RP, Smith KT, Recker RR, Hinders SM. Meal effects on calcium absorption. *Am J Clin Nutr.* 1989 Feb;49(2):372-6.

227 *Department of Human Services Healthy Guidelines for Americans,* 2000.

228 Hilton E, Isenberg HD, Alperstein P, France K, Borenstein MT. Ingestion of yogurt containing Lactobacillus acidophilus as prophylaxis for candidal vaginitis. *Ann Intern Med.* 1992 Mar 1;116(5):353-7.

229 Whysner J, Williams GM. Saccharin mechanistic data and risk assessment: urine composition, enhanced cell proliferation, and tumor promotion. *Pharmacol Ther.* 1996;71(1-2):225-52.

230 Cohen SM, Arnold LL, Cano M, Ito M, Garland EM, Shaw RA. Calcium phosphate-containing precipitate and the carcinogenicity of sodium salts in rats. *Carcinogenesis.* 2000 Apr;21(4):783-92.

231 Cohen SM. Role of urinary physiology and chemistry in bladder carcinogenesis. *Food Chem Toxicol.* 1995 Sep;33(9):715-30.

232 Aspartame. Review of safety issues. Council on Scientific Affairs. *JAMA.* 1985 Jul 19;254(3):400-2.

233 Weihrauch MR, Diehl V. Artificial sweeteners—do they bear a carcinogenic risk? *Ann Oncol.* 2004 Oct;15(10):1460-5.

234 Alcohol-attributable deaths and years of potential life lost—United States, 2001. *MMWR Morb Mortal Wkly Rep.* 2004 Sep 24;53(37):866-70.

235 Thomas DB. Alcohol as a cause of cancer. *Environ Health Perspect.* 1995 Nov;103 Suppl 8:153-60.

236 *American Heart Association Eating Plan for Healthy Americans,* 2000.

237 Klatsky AL, Friedman GD, Armstrong MA, Kipp H. Wine, liquor, beer, and mortality. *Am J Epidemiol.* 2003 Sep 15;158(6):585-95.

238 Mukamal KJ, Conigrave KM, Mittleman MA, Camargo CA Jr, Stampfer MJ, Willett WC, Rimm EB. Roles of drinking pattern and type of alcohol consumed in coronary heart disease in men. *N Engl J Med.* 2003 Jan 9;348(2):109-18.

239 Renaud S, Lanzmann-Petithory D, Gueguen R, Conard P. Alcohol and mortality from all causes. *Biol Res.* 2004;37(2):183-7.

240 Mukamal KJ, Conigrave KM, Mittleman MA, Camargo CA Jr, Stampfer MJ, Willett WC, Rimm EB. Roles of drinking pattern and type of alcohol consumed in coronary heart disease in men. *N Engl J Med.* 2003 Jan 9;348(2):109-18.

241 Mukamal KJ, Kuller LH, Fitzpatrick AL, Longstreth WT Jr, Mittleman MA, Siscovick DS. Prospective study of alcohol consumption and risk of dementia in older adults. *JAMA.* 2003 Mar 19;289(11):1405-13.

242 Ruitenberg A, van Swieten JC, Witteman JC, Mehta KM, van Duijn CM, Hofman A, Breteler MM. Alcohol consumption and risk of dementia: the Rotterdam Study. *Lancet.* 2002 Jan 26;359(9303):281-6.

243 Yang CS, Landau JM, Huang MT, Newmark HL. Inhibition of carcinogenesis by dietary polyphenolic compounds. *Annu Rev Nutr.* 2001;21:381-406.

244 Hannigan JH, Armant DR. Alcohol in pregnancy and neonatal outcome. *Semin Neonatol.* 2000 Aug;5(3):243-54.

245 Mennella J. Alcohol's effect on lactation. *Alcohol Res Health.* 2001;25(3):230-4.

246 Prevention of Pediatric Overweight and Obesity, *Pediatrics.* 2003;112:424-430

247 Hammer LD, Kraemer HC, Wilson DM, Ritter PL, Dornbusch SM. Standardized percentile curves of body-mass index for children and adolescents. *Am J Dis Child.* 1991 Mar;145(3):259-63.

248 Yanovski JA. Pediatric obesity. *Rev Endocr Metab Disord.* 2001 Oct;2(4):371-83.

249 Ogden CL. Defining overweight in children using growth charts. *Md Med.* 2004 Summer;5(3):19-21.

250 Hedley AA, Ogden CL, Johnson CL, Carroll MD, Curtin LR, Flegal KM. Prevalence of overweight and obesity among US children, adolescents, and adults, 1999-2002. *JAMA.* 2004 Jun 16;291(23):2847-50.

251 Galtier-Dereure F, Boegner C, Bringer J. Obesity and pregnancy: complications and cost. *Am J Clin Nutr.* 2000 May;71(5 Suppl):1242S-8S.

252 Streissguth AP, Aase JM, Clarren SK, Randels SP, LaDue RA, Smith DF. Fetal alcohol syndrome in adolescents and adults. *JAMA.* 1991 Apr 17;265(15):1961-7.

253 Spohr HL, Willms J, Steinhausen HC. Prenatal alcohol exposure and long-term developmental consequences. Lancet. 1993 Apr 10;341(8850):907-10.

254 Day NL, Zuo Y, Richardson GA, Goldschmidt L, Larkby CA, Cornelius MD. Prenatal alcohol use and offspring size at 10 years of age. *Alcohol Clin Exp Res*. 1999 May;23(5):863-9.

255 Olson HC, Feldman JJ, Streissguth AP, Sampson PD, Bookstein FL. Neuropsychological deficits in adolescents with fetal alcohol syndrome: clinical findings. *Alcohol Clin Exp Res*. 1998 Dec;22(9):1998-2012.

256 Streissguth AP, Barr HM, Sampson PD. Moderate prenatal alcohol exposure: effects on child IQ and learning problems at age 7 1/2 years. *Alcohol Clin Exp Res*. 1990 Oct;14(5):662-9.

257 Prevention of neural tube defects: results of the Medical Research Council Vitamin Study. MRC Vitamin Study Research Group. Lancet. 1991 Jul 20;338(8760):131-7.

258 Centers for Disease Control and Prevention (CDC). Spina bifida and anencephaly before and after folic acid mandate—United States, 1995-1996 and 1999-2000. MMWR *Morb Mortal Wkly Rep*. 2004 May 7;53(17):362-5.

259 Wald NJ, Law MR, Morris JK, Wald DS. Quantifying the effect of folic acid. *Lancet*. 2001 Dec 15;358(9298):2069-73.

260 Wilson RD, Davies G, Desilets V, Reid GJ, Summers A, Wyatt P, Young D; Genetics Committee and Executive and Council of the Society of Obstetricians and Gynaecologists of Canada. The use of folic acid for the prevention of neural tube defects and other congenital anomalies. *J Obstet Gynaecol Can*. 2003 Nov;25(11):959-73.

261 Gartner LM, Morton J, Lawrence RA, Naylor AJ, O'Hare D, Schanler RJ, Eidelman AI; American Academy of Pediatrics Section on Breastfeeding. Breastfeeding and the use of human milk. *Pediatrics*. 2005 Feb;115(2):496-506.

262 Must A, Spadano J, Coakley EH, Field AE, Colditz G, Dietz WH. The disease burden associated with overweight and obesity. JAMA. 1999 Oct 27;282(16):1523-9.

263 Williamson DF, Vinicor F, Bowman BA; Centers For Disease Control And Prevention Primary Prevention Working Group. Primary prevention of type 2 diabetes mellitus by lifestyle intervention: implications for health policy. Ann Intern Med. 2004 Jun 1;140(11):951-7.

264 Nutrition Principles and Recommendations in Diabetes. *Diabetes Care* 27:S36, 2004.

265 Sasco AJ, Secretan MB, Straif K. Tobacco smoking and cancer: a brief review of recent epidemiological evidence. *Lung Cancer*. 2004 Aug;45 Suppl 2:S3-9.

266 Burns DM. Epidemiology of smoking-induced cardiovascular disease. *Prog Cardiovasc Dis*. 2003 Jul-Aug;46(1):11-29.

267 *The Practical Guide Identification, Evaluation, and Treatment of Overweight and Obesity in Adults*, National Heart, Lung, and Blood Institute and North American Association for the Study of Obesity, 2000.

268 Gebhart SE, Thomas RG. Nutritive Value of Foods. *Home and Garden Bulletin* Number 72, United States Department of Agriculture, Agricultural Research Service, 2002.

269 Avenell A, Brown TJ, McGee MA, Campbell MK, Grant AM, Broom J, Jung RT, Smith WC. What interventions should we add to weight reducing diets in adults with obesity? A systematic review of randomized controlled trials of adding drug therapy, exercise, behaviour therapy or combinations of these interventions. *J Hum Nutr Diet*. 2004 Aug;17(4):293-316.

270 Slentz CA, Duscha BD, Johnson JL, Ketchum K, Aiken LB, Samsa GP, Houmard JA, Bales CW, Kraus WE. Effects of the amount of exercise on body weight, body composition, and measures of central obesity: STRRIDE—a randomized controlled study. *Arch Intern Med*. 2004 Jan 12;164(1):31-9.

271 Press V, Freestone I, George CF. Physical activity: the evidence of benefit in the prevention of coronary heart disease. QJM. 2003 Apr;96(4):245-51.

272 Morris JN, Everitt MG, Pollard R, Chave SP, Semmence AM. Vigorous exercise in leisure-time: protection against coronary heart disease. *Lancet*. 1980 Dec 6;2(8206):1207-10.

273 Lee IM, Hsieh CC, Paffenbarger RS Jr. Exercise intensity and longevity in men. The Harvard Alumni Health Study. JAMA. 1995 Apr 19;273(15):1179-84.

274 Saris WH, Blair SN, van Baak MA, Eaton SB, Davies PS, Di Pietro L, Fogelholm M, Rissanen A, Schoeller D, Swinburn B, Tremblay A, Westerterp KR, Wyatt H. How much physical activity is enough to prevent unhealthy weight gain? Outcome of the IASO 1st Stock Conference and consensus statement. *Obes Rev*. 2003 May;4(2):101-14.

275 George BJ, Goldberg N. The benefits of exercise in geriatric women. *Am J Geriatr Cardiol*. 2001 Sep-Oct;10(5):260-3.

276 Sherman SE, D'Agostino RB, Cobb JL, Kannel WB. Does exercise reduce mortality rates in the elderly? Experience from the Framingham Heart Study. *Am Heart J*. 1994 Nov;128(5):965-72.

277 Jolliffe JA, Rees K, Taylor RS, Thompson D, Oldridge N, Ebrahim S. Exercise-based rehabilitation for coronary heart disease. *Cochrane Database Syst Rev*. 2001;(1):CD001800.

278 American Heart Association web site.

279 *The Practical Guide Identification, Evaluation, and Treatment of Overweight and Obesity in Adults*, National Heart, Lung, and Blood Institute and North American Association for the Study of Obesity, 2000.

280 Byrne SM. Psychological aspects of weight maintenance and relapse in obesity. *J Psychosom Res*. 2002 Nov;53(5):1029-36.

281 Blundell JE, Gillett A. Control of food intake in the obese. *Obes Res*. 2001 Nov;9 Suppl 4:263S-270S.

282 Laitinen J, Ek E, Sovio U. Stress-related eating and drinking behavior and body mass index and predictors of this behavior. *Prev Med*. 2002 Jan;34(1):29-39.

283 Vanderlinden J, Dalla Grave R, Vandereycken W, Noorduin C. Which factors do provoke binge-eating? An exploratory study in female students. *Eat Behav*. 2001 Spring;2(1):79-83.

284 Johnston E, Johnson S, McLeod P, Johnston M. The relation of body mass index to depressive symptoms. *Can J Public Health*. 2004 May-Jun;95(3):179-83.

285 Jain AK, Kaplan RA, Gadde KM, Wadden TA, Allison DB, Brewer ER, Leadbetter RA, Richard N, Haight B, Jamerson BD, Buaron KS, Metz A. Bupropion SR vs. placebo for weight loss in obese patients with depressive symptoms. *Obes Res*. 2002 Oct;10(10):1049-56.

286 Berteus Forslund H, Torgerson JS, Sjostrom L, Lindroos AK. Snacking frequency in relation to energy intake and food choices in obese men and women compared to a reference population. *Int J Obes Relat Metab Disord*. 2005 Jun;29(6):711-9.

287 Berteus Forslund H, Lindroos AK, Sjostrom L, Lissner L. Meal patterns and obesity in Swedish women-a simple instrument describing usual meal types, frequency and temporal distribution. *Eur J Clin Nutr*. 2002 Aug;56(8):740-7.

288 Vorona RD, Winn MP, Babineau TW, Eng BP, Feldman HR, Ware JC. Overweight and obese patients in a primary care population report less sleep than patients with a normal body mass index. *Arch Intern Med*. 2005 Jan 10;165(1):25-30.

289 Taheri S, Lin L, Austin D, Young T, Mignot E. Short sleep duration is associated with reduced leptin, elevated ghrelin, and increased body mass index. *PLoS Med*. 2004 Dec;1(3):e62.

290 Badman MK, Flier JS. *The gut and energy balance: visceral allies in the obesity wars*. Science. 2005 Mar 25;307(5717):1909-14.

291 Banks WA. The many lives of leptin. *Peptides*. 2004 Mar;25(3):331-8.

292 Spiegelman BM, Flier JS. Obesity and the regulation of energy balance. *Cell*. 2001 Feb 23;104(4):531-43.

293 Ariyasu H, Takaya K, Tagami T, Ogawa Y, Hosoda K, Akamizu T, Suda M, Koh T, Natsui K, Toyooka S, Shirakami G, Usui T, Shimatsu A, Doi K, Hosoda H, Kojima M, Kangawa K, Nakao K. Stomach is a major source of circulating ghrelin, and feeding state determines plasma ghrelin-like immunoreactivity levels in humans. *J Clin Endocrinol Metab*. 2001 Oct;86(10):4753-8.

294 Banks WA, Tschop M, Robinson SM, Heiman ML. Extent and direction of ghrelin transport across the blood-brain barrier is determined by its unique primary structure. *J Pharmacol Exp Ther*. 2002 Aug;302(2):822-7.

295 Wren AM, Seal LJ, Cohen MA, Brynes AE, Frost GS, Murphy KG, Dhillo WS, Ghatei MA, Bloom SR. Ghrelin enhances appetite and increases food intake in humans. *J Clin Endocrinol Metab*. 2001 Dec;86(12):5992.

296 Samson WK, Taylor MM, Ferguson AV. Non-sleep effects of hypocretin/orexin. *Sleep Med Rev*. 2005 Aug;9(4):243-52.

297 Prospero-Garcia O, Mendez-Diaz M. The role of neuropeptides in sleep modulation. *Drug News Perspect*. 2004 Oct;17(8):518-22.

298 Weikel JC, Wichniak A, Ising M, Brunner H, Friess E, Held K, Mathias S, Schmid DA, Uhr M, Steiger A. Ghrelin promotes slow-wave sleep in humans. *Am J Physiol Endocrinol Metab*. 2003 Feb;284(2):E407-15.

299 Taheri S, Lin L, Austin D, Young T, Mignot E. Short sleep duration is associated with reduced leptin, elevated ghrelin, and increased body mass index. *PLoS Med*. 2004 Dec;1(3):e62. Epub 2004 Dec 7.

300 Eating Disorders: Facts About Eating Disorders and the Search for Solutions, National Institute of Mental Health, 2000.

301 Herzog DB, Nussbaum KM, Marmor AK. Comorbidity and outcome in eating disorders. *Psychiatr Clin North Am*. 1996 Dec;19(4):843-59.

302 Hoek HW, van Hoeken D. Review of the prevalence and incidence of eating disorders. *Int J Eat Disord*. 2003 Dec;34(4):383-96.

303 American Psychiatric Association, *Diagnostic and Statistical Manual of Mental Disorders: DSM-IV*, American Psychiatric Press, 1994, pp. 539-545.

304 Nielsen S, Moller-Madsen S, Isager T, Jorgensen J, Pagsberg K, Theander S. Standardized mortality in eating disorders—a quantitative summary of previously published and new evidence. *J Psychosom Res*. 1998 Mar-Apr;44(3-4):413-34.

305 Sullivan PF. Mortality in anorexia nervosa. *Am J Psychiatry*. 1995 Jul;152(7):1073-4.

306 Pompili M, Mancinelli I, Girardi P, Ruberto A, Tatarelli R. Suicide in anorexia nervosa: A meta-analysis. *Int J Eat Disord*. 2004 Jul;36(1):99-103.

307 Keel PK, Dorer DJ, Eddy KT, Franko D, Charatan DL, Herzog DB. Predictors of mortality in eating disorders. *Arch Gen Psychiatry*. 2003 Feb;60(2):179-83.

308 Hoek HW, van Hoeken D. Review of the prevalence and incidence of eating disorders. *Int J Eat Disord*. 2003 Dec;34(4):383-96.

309 American Psychiatric Association, *Diagnostic and Statistical Manual of Mental Disorders: DSM-IV*, American Psychiatric Press, 1994, pp. 545-550.

310 Hoek HW, van Hoeken D. Review of the prevalence and incidence of eating disorders. *Int J Eat Disord*. 2003 Dec;34(4):383-96.

311 American Psychiatric Association, *Diagnostic and Statistical Manual of Mental Disorders: DSM-IV*, American Psychiatric Press, 1994, pp. 729-731.

312 Lloyd-Richardson EE, King TK, Forsyth LH, Clark MM. Body image evaluations in obese females with binge eating disorder. *Eat Behav*. 2000 Dec;1(2):161-71.

313 Dingemans AE, Bruna MJ, van Furth EF. Binge eating disorder: a review. *Int J Obes Relat Metab Disord*. 2002 Mar;26(3):299-307.

314 Rand CS, Macgregor AM, Stunkard AJ. The night eating syndrome in the general population and among postoperative obesity surgery patients. *Int J Eat Disord*. 1997 Jul;22(1):65-9.

315 Adami GE, Meneghelli A, Scopinaro N. Night eating syndrome in individuals with Mediterranean eating-style. *Eat Weight Disord*. 1997 Dec;2(4):203-6.

316 Spaggiari MC, Granella F, Parrino L, Marchesi C, Melli I, Terzano MG. Nocturnal eating syndrome in adults. *Sleep*. 1994 Jun;17(4):339-44.

317 Winkelman JW. Clinical and polysomnographic features of sleep-related eating disorder. *J Clin Psychiatry*. 1998 Jan;59(1):14-9.

318 Gluck ME, Geliebter A, Satov T. Night eating syndrome is associated with depression, low self-esteem, reduced daytime hunger, and less weight loss in obese outpatients. *Obes Res*. 2001 Apr;9(4):264-7.

319 O'Reardon JP, Stunkard AJ, Allison KC. Clinical trial of sertraline in the treatment of night eating syndrome. *Int J Eat Disord*. 2004 Jan;35(1):16-26.

320 James WPT, Astrup Al, Finer N, et al. Effect of sibutramine on weight maintenance after weight loss: a randomised trial. *Lancet.* 2000;356:2119-2125.

321 Arterburn DE, Crane PK, Veenstra DL. The efficacy and safety of sibutramine for weight loss: a systematic review. *Arch Intern Med.* 2004 May 10;164(9):994-1003.

322 Davidson MH, Hauptman J, DiGirolamo M, Foreyt JP, Halsted CH, Heber D, Heimburger DC, Lucas CP, Robbins DC, Chung J, Heymsfield SB. Weight control and risk factor reduction in obese subjects treated for 2 years with orlistat: a randomized controlled trial. *JAMA.* 1999 Jan 20;281(3):235-42.

323 Foxcroft DR, Milne R. Orlistat for the treatment of obesity: rapid review and cost-effectiveness model. *Obes Rev.* 2000 Oct;1(2):121-6.

324 Haller CA, Benowitz NL. Adverse cardiovascular and central nervous system events associated with dietary supplements containing ephedra alkaloids. *N Engl J Med.* 2000 Dec 21;343(25):1833-8.

325 Rampton S, Stauber, J. Swallowing Anything: The Hype Behind Alternative Remedies. *PR Watch.* 1997; 4(3):1-5.

326 Maggard MA, Shugarman LR, Suttorp M, Maglione M, Sugarman HJ, Livingston EH, Nguyen NT, Li Z, Mojica WA, Hilton L, Rhodes S, Morton SC, Shekelle PG. Meta-analysis: surgical treatment of obesity. *Ann Intern Med.* 2005 Apr 5;142(7):547-59.

327 Sugerman HJ. Bariatric surgery for severe obesity. *J Assoc Acad Minor Phys.* 2001 Jul;12(3):129-36.

328 Maggard MA, Shugarman LR, Suttorp M, Maglione M, Sugarman HJ, Livingston EH, Nguyen NT, Li Z, Mojica WA, Hilton L, Rhodes S, Morton SC, Shekelle PG. Meta-analysis: surgical treatment of obesity. *Ann Intern Med.* 2005 Apr 5;142(7):547-59.

329 Fernandez AZ Jr, Demaria EJ, Tichansky DS, Kellum JM, Wolfe LG, Meador J, Sugerman HJ. Multivariate analysis of risk factors for death following gastric bypass for treatment of morbid obesity. *Ann Surg.* 2004 May;239(5):698-702.

330 Dymek MP, le Grange D, Neven K, Alverdy J. Quality of life and psychosocial adjustment in patients after Roux-en-Y gastric bypass: a brief report. *Obes Surg.* 2001 Feb;11(1):32-9.

331 Hafner RJ, Rogers J. Husbands' adjustment to wives' weight loss after gastric restriction for morbid obesity. *Int J Obes.* 1990 Dec;14(12):1069-78.

332 Hafner RJ, Watts JM, Rogers J. Quality of life after gastric bypass for morbid obesity. *Int J Obes.* 1991 Aug;15(8):555-60.

333 Fernandez AZ Jr, Demaria EJ, Tichansky DS, Kellum JM, Wolfe LG, Meador J, Sugerman HJ. Multivariate analysis of risk factors for death following gastric bypass for treatment of morbid obesity. *Ann Surg.* 2004 May;239(5):698-702.

334 Smith SC, Edwards CB, Goodman GN, Halversen RC, Simper SC. Open vs laparoscopic Roux-en-Y gastric bypass: comparison of operative morbidity and mortality. *Obes Surg.* 2004 Jan;14(1):73-6.

335 Courcoulas A, Perry Y, Buenaventura P, Luketich J. Comparing the outcomes after laparoscopic versus open gastric bypass: a matched paired analysis. *Obes Surg.* 2003 Jun;13(3):341-6.

336 Fernandez AZ Jr, DeMaria EJ, Tichansky DS, Kellum JM, Wolfe LG, Meador J, Sugerman HJ. Experience with over 3,000 open and laparoscopic bariatric procedures: multivariate analysis of factors related to leak and resultant mortality. *Surg Endosc.* 2004 Feb;18(2):193-7.

337 Lee WB, Hamilton SM, Harris JP, Schwab IR. Ocular complications of hypovitaminosis A after bariatric surgery. *Ophthalmology.* 2005 May.

338 Gebhart SE, Thomas RG. Nutritive Value of Foods. *Home and Garden Bulletin* Number 72, United States Department of Agriculture, Agricultural Research Service, 2002.

339 United States Department of Agriculture, Human Nutrition Information Service, *Home and Garden Bulletin* Number 250, 1993.

340 *2005 Dietary Guidelines Report*, United States Department of Health and Human Services and United States Department of Agriculture.

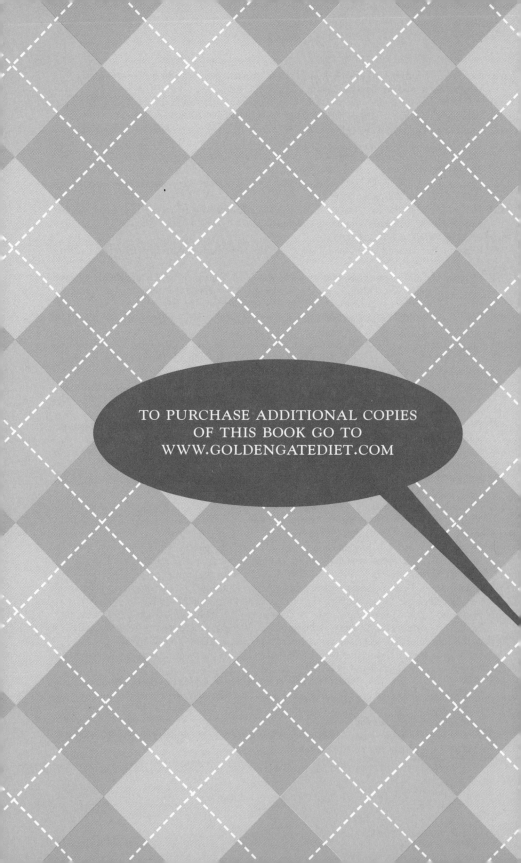

TO PURCHASE ADDITIONAL COPIES
OF THIS BOOK GO TO
WWW.GOLDENGATEDIET.COM